Pocket Picture Guides

Lipids and Lipid Disorders

An **Essential Slide Collection of Lipids and Lipid Disorders**, based on the contents of this book, is available. The collection consists of numbered 35 mm colour transparencies of each illustration in the book, and each section is accompanied by a slide index for easy reference. The material is presented in an attractive binder, which also contains a copy of the Pocket Picture Guide. The Essential Slide Collection is available from:

Mosby–Year Book Europe Limited

Lynton House,
7–12 Tavistock Square,
London WC1H 9LB, UK

Pocket Picture Guides

Lipids and Lipid Disorders

Michael D. Feher
MB BS, MRCP

Lecturer
Department of Clinical Pharmacology and Therapeutics
Charing Cross and Westminster Medical School
London, UK

William Richmond
PhD

Top Grade Biochemist
Diagnostic Chemical Pathology
St Mary's Hospital
London, UK

ℳ Wolfe

Publisher: Fiona Foley
Project Editor: Alison Whitehouse
Design: Olgun Hassan
              Richard Prime
              Patrizia Cavaliere
              John Codling

Illustration: Marie McNestry
Production: Susan Bishop
Index: Nina Boyd

Library of Congress Cataloging-in-Publication Data
Feher, Michael D.
Pocket picture guides: lipids and lipid disorders/Michael D. Feher,
William
Richmond.
Includes index.
1. Lipids—Metabolism—Disorders—Atlases. I. Richmond, William.
II. Title.
RC623,L5F44 1990
616.3'997—dc20

Typesetting by Tradespools Ltd, Frome, Somerset
Text set in Sabon; captions and figures set in Frutiger.
Produced by Mandarin Offset
Printed by Mandarin Offset Ltd, Hong Kong

Copyright © 1991 Gower Medical Publishing
Published in 1991 by Gower Medical Publishing
Reprinted in 1994 by Wolfe Publishing, an imprint of Mosby–Year Book
Europe Ltd, Lynton House, 7–12 Tavistock Square, London WC1H
9LB, England.
ISBN 0 397 44685 3

For full details of all Mosby–Year Book Europe Limited titles please
write to Mosby–Year Book Europe Limited, Lynton House, 7–12
Tavistock Square, London WC1H 9LB, England.

A CIP catalogue record for this book is available from the British
Library.

PREFACE

In recent years, increasing awareness of the impact of lipid disorders on clinical disease has focused attention on the complexity of the underlying biochemistry and the epidemiology of these conditions. Consequently, there have been many advances in the understanding of genetic and environmental influences on lipoprotein metabolism, and in the development of effective guidelines for dietary and drug therapy. We hope that this Pocket Picture Guide presents an accessible summary of this complex field, and fulfils its aim of providing both a theoretical background and a practical guide to the investigation and management of patients with lipid disorders.

We are grateful to our many clinical and research colleagues who have stimulated our interest in this field and provided us with an enjoyable work arena in this challenging and exciting area of medicine.

Michael D. Feher
William Richmond

London, July 1990

ACKNOWLEDGEMENTS

The authors would like to thank the following colleagues for providing illustrative material: Professor A. F. Lant, London (Figs 38 & 39); Dr R. S. Elkeles, London (Figs 43 & 44); Dr D. Leslie, London (Fig. 55); Dr A. F. Branfoot, London (Fig. 59); Dr A. D. Timmis, London (Fig. 55), Dr J. Gleeson (Figs 56 & 57).

The assistance of the Departments of Medical Illustration, St Mary's Hospital, Charing Cross and Westminster Medical Schools, London, is gratefully acknowledged.

ABBREVIATIONS AND UNITS

ATML	adipose tissue mobilizing lipase
ACAT	acyl:cholesterol acyltransferase
ACE	angiotensin converting enzyme
apo A	apolipoprotein A
apo B	apolipoprotein B
apo C	apolipoprotein C
apo D	apolipoprotein D
apo E	apolipoprotein E
CE	cholesterol ester
CETP	cholesterol ester transferase protein
CHD	coronary heart disease
CHYLO	chylomicron
d	density
FC	free cholesterol
FFA	free fatty acid
FH	familial hypercholesterolaemia
γ*GT*	gamma-glutamyl transpeptidase
HDL	high-density lipoprotein
HMG	β-hydroxy-β-
CoA	methylglutaryl-coenzyme A
HTGL	hepatic triglyceride lipase
IDDM	insulin-dependent (type 1) diabetes mellitus
IDL	intermediate-density lipoprotein
IHD	ischaemic heart disease
LCAT	lecithin: cholesterol acyltransferase
Lp(a)	lipoprotein (a)
LDL	low density lipoprotein
NIDDM	non-insulin-dependent (type 2) diabetes mellitus
OH	hydroxyl
TC	total cholesterol
TG	triglyceride
VLDL	very low density lipoprotein

CONVERSION OF CHOLESTEROL AND TRIGLYCERIDE VALUES

mg/dl cholesterol = mmol/l $\times$ 38.6

mg/dl triglyceride = mmol/l $\times$ 88.5

CHOLESTEROL

mg/dl	mmol/l
500	12
400	10
300	8
	6
200	4
100	2
0	0

TRIGLYCERIDE

mg/dl	mmol/l
	15
1200	
1000	10
800	
600	
400	5
200	
0	0

CONTENTS

LIPIDS: CHEMISTRY AND CLASSIFICATION

Lipids are water-insoluble organic molecules characterized by the hydrocarbon nature of a major portion of their structure.

Simple lipids

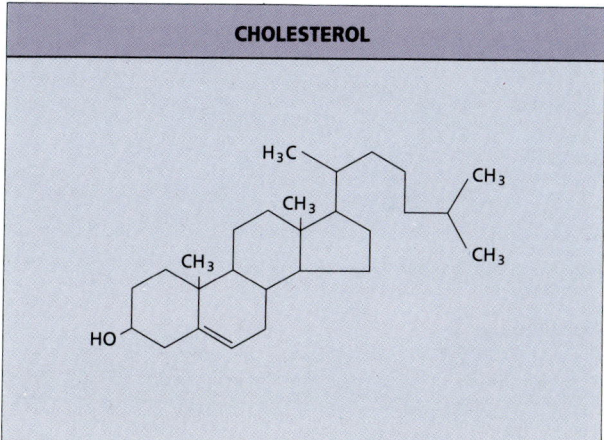

CHOLESTEROL

Fig. 1 Cholesterol, a steroid alcohol, is a key structural component of membranes in animal tissues, and a precursor of many other steroids including bile acids and steroid hormones.

FATTY ACIDS	
type	**hydrocarbon chain**
saturated	containing no double bonds
monounsaturated	containing one double bond
polyunsaturated	containing two or more double bonds

Fig. 2 Fatty acids.

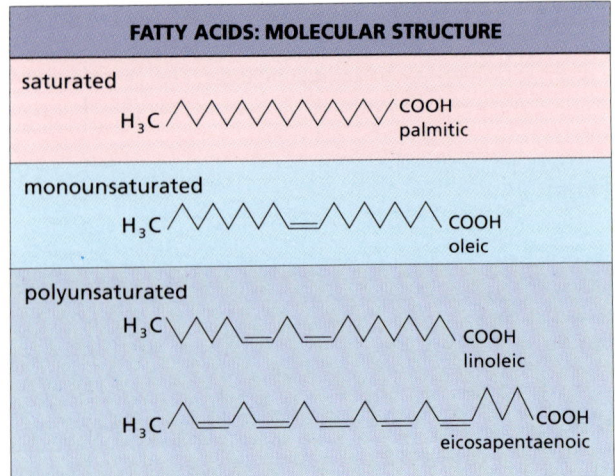

Fig. 3 Examples of fatty acids.

FATTY ACIDS: NOMENCLATURE AND SOURCES			
fatty acid	family	nomenclature	main dietary source
palmitic	saturated	16:0	animal fat
oleic	$\omega-9$	$18:1,\omega-9$	vegetable oils
linoleic	$\omega-6$	$18:2,\omega-6$	vegetable oils
eicosapentaenoic	$\omega-3$	$20:5,\omega-3$	fish oils

Fig. 4 Fatty acids are described by a nomenclature that indicates:
The number of carbon atoms in the molecule: **xx**:x,ω−x.
The number of double bonds: xx:**x**,ω−x.
The position of the first double bond counting from the terminal (ω) carbon atom: xx:x,ω−**x**.

Fatty acids are an important energy source and are integral components of complex lipids. Essential fatty acids, such as linoleic acid, cannot be synthesized by mammals and are required in the diet as precursors for prostaglandin synthesis.

Complex lipids

Complex lipids are produced when fatty acids (FA) combine with molecules containing alcohol (−OH) groups to form esters. The major complex lipids in plasma are cholesterol esters and glycerol esters.

Cholesterol esters

Cholesterol is relatively polar as the free alcohol but non-polar when esterified. A large proportion (75%) of plasma cholesterol is esterified. The most abundant in human plasma are cholesterol linoleate (43%) and cholesterol oleate (24%).

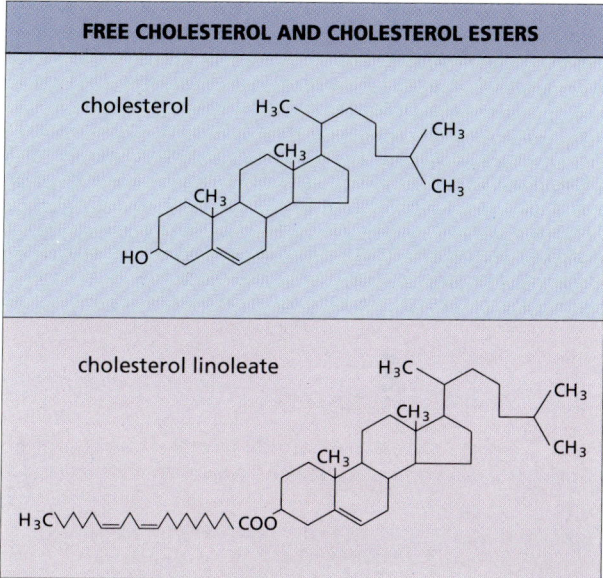

FREE CHOLESTEROL AND CHOLESTEROL ESTERS

cholesterol

cholesterol linoleate

Fig. 5 Cholesterol esters.

Glycerol esters: triglycerides and phospholipids

When all three hydroxyl groups of glycerol are esterified with fatty acids the molecule becomes very non-polar and is called a triacylglycerol or triglyceride. Triglycerides (TGs) are stored in adipose tissue and represent an energy source from which fatty acids can be released during periods of starvation.

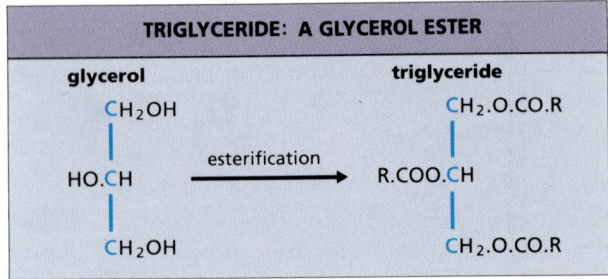

Fig. 6 Triglyceride results from esterification of glycerol with fatty acids. R = carbon chain of fatty acids.

Phosphoglycerides, a class of phospholipids, differ from triglycerides in that the terminal hydroxyl groups of glycerol are esterified to phosphate-containing molecules rather than fatty acids.

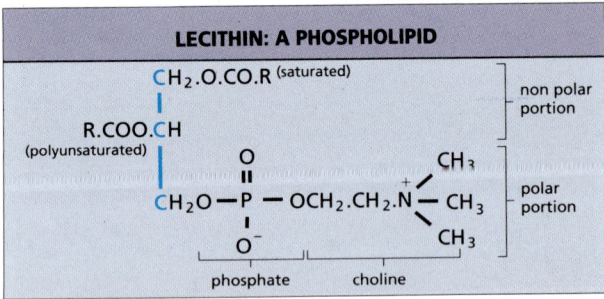

Fig. 7 Lecithin incorporates choline phosphate and is an example of an important phospholipid. R = carbon chain of fatty acids.

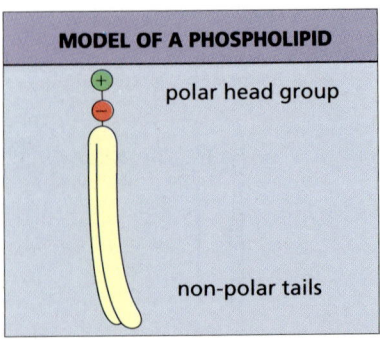

Fig. 8 Model of a phospholipid. Possession of a polar phosphate ester head group, together with non-polar hydrocarbon tails, enables phospholipids to play an important structural role in cell membranes and lipoprotein complexes.[1]

LIPOPROTEINS: STRUCTURE AND FUNCTION

Lipoproteins

Lipids, being insoluble in aqueous solution, are transported in plasma in association with specialized proteins, apolipoproteins (apoproteins) in spherical lipoprotein complexes. *Apoproteins* possess helical regions that are amphipathic; one surface of the helix contains hydrophobic amino acid residues while the other is hydrophilic. This enables apoproteins to bind phospholipid by hydrophobic interaction.

In lipoprotein structures the polar head groups of phospholipids and the alcohol groups of unesterified cholesterol project from the surface of the particle into the aqueous environment. The non-polar portions of these molecules project into the core of the particle which contains non-polar cholesterol esters (CE) and triglyceride. Amphipathic apoproteins complete the membrane-like surface of the structure by binding phospholipid and interacting with the aqueous environment and the lipid core.

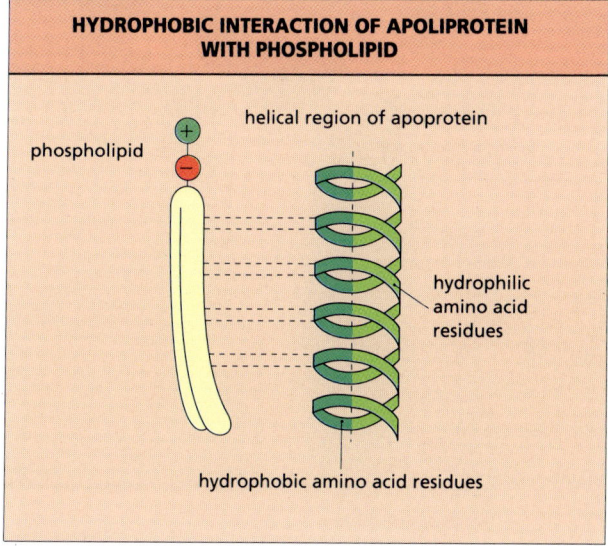

Fig. 9 Hydrophobic interaction of apolipoprotein with phospholipid.[1]

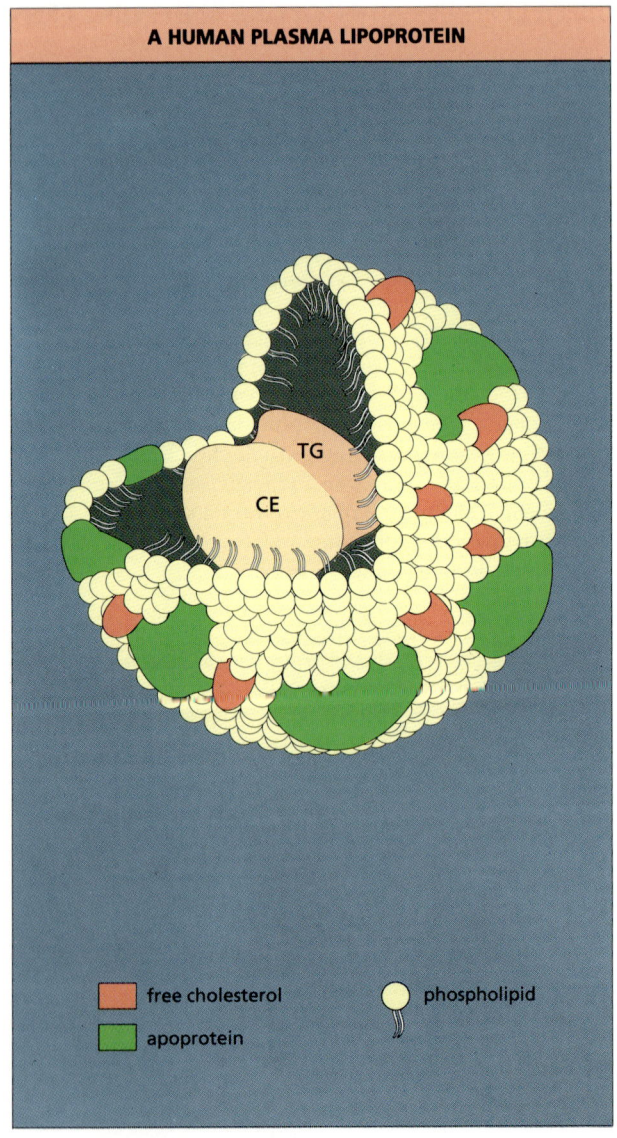

Fig. 10 A plasma lipoprotein.

The plasma lipoproteins

The plasma lipoproteins have been fractionated by ultracentrifugation into five major density classes—density is conferred by the proportion of protein in the complexes. The distribution of lipids and apoproteins differs between classes, and the particles differ in size and electrophoretic mobility. Each lipoprotein class is heterogeneous in composition. For example, HDL can be sub-fractionated into HDL3 ($d = 1.125$–1.210 g/ml) and HDL2 ($d = 1.063$–1.125 g/ml), a larger particle with a greater lipid load.

The main cholesterol-carrying lipoproteins are LDL and HDL. In a normal individual, LDL contains approximately 70% and HDL 20% of the total plasma cholesterol.

The main triglyceride-carrying lipoproteins are chylomicrons and VLDLs. Chylomicrons are not normally present in blood after a 12 h fast. In the fasting state VLDLs account for approximately 60% of the total plasma triglyceride.

THE DENSITY CLASSES OF PLASMA LIPOPROTEINS				
	density (*d*; g/ml)	sources	electrophoretic mobility	mean diameter (nm)
chylomicrons CHYLO	<0.95	intestine	origin	500
very low density lipoproteins VLDL	<1.006	liver	pre-β	43
intermediate density lipoproteins IDL	1.006–1.019	catabolism of VLDL & chylomicrons	'broad β'	27
low density lipoprotein LDL	1.019–1.063	catabolism of VLDL	β	22
high density lipoproteins HDL	1.063–1.21	catabolism of chylomicrons & VLDL; liver & intestine	α	8

Fig. 11   The five major density classes of lipoproteins.

COMPOSITION OF THE PLASMA LIPOPROTEINS					
	CHYLO	VLDL	IDL	LDL	HDL
protein	2	10	18	25	55
triglyceride	85	50	26	10	4
cholesterol	1	7	12	8	2
cholesterol ester	3	13	22	37	15
phospholipid	9	20	22	20	24

Fig. 12 Composition of the plasma lipoproteins (% total).

APOPROTEIN DISTRIBUTION IN LIPOPROTEIN CLASSES					
	CHYLO	VLDL	IDL	LDL	HDL
apoproteins (major)	C-III	B-100	B-100	B-100	A-I
	C-II	C-III	B-48*		A-II
	C-I	E	E		D
	B-48	C-II			C-III
	E	C-I			C-I
	A-I	A-I			E
(minor)	A-II	A-II			
*Chylomicron remnants only.					

Fig. 13 Apoprotein distribution in lipoprotein classes.

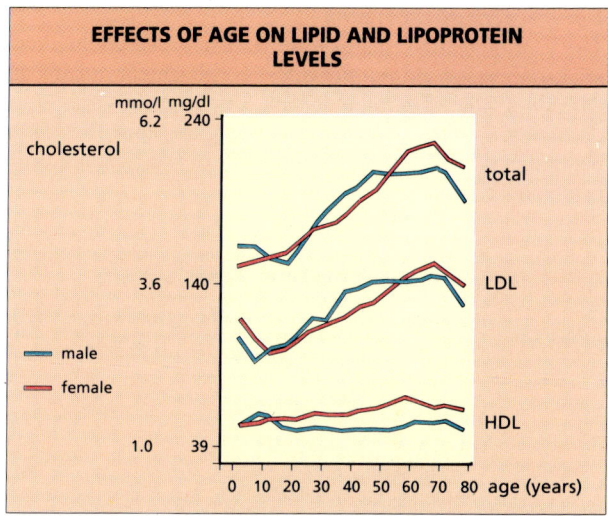

Fig. 14 Mean plasma levels of total, LDL and HDL cholesterol in men and women at different ages.

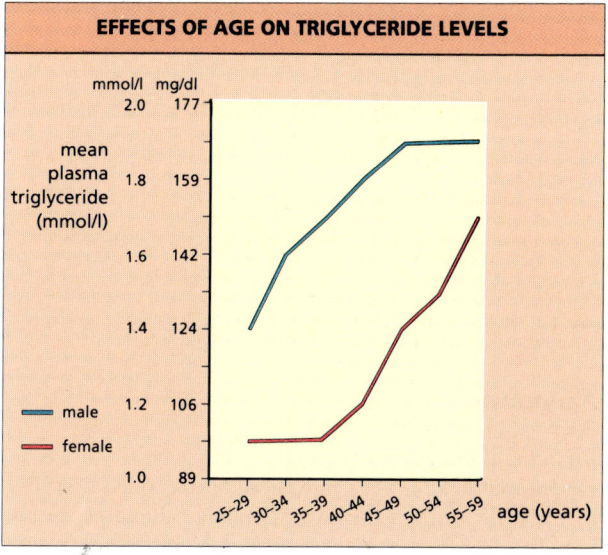

Fig. 15 Fasting plasma triglyceride concentrations in men and women at different ages.[2]

Lipoprotein phenotyping

The World Health Organization system, based on the Frederickson classification, provides a convenient means of describing the lipoprotein profile of the most commonly occurring patterns of hyperlipidaemia, the lipid elevations being determined by the composition of the elevated lipoprotein fractions.

PHENOTYPING OF HYPERLIPOPROTEINAEMIAS			
phenotype	lipoprotein abnormality	major plasma lipid elevation	minor plasma lipid elevation
I	chylomicrons	triglycerides	cholesterol
IIa	LDL (β)	cholesterol	
IIb	LDL (β) and VLDL (pre-β)	cholesterol and triglycerides	
III	IDL (β)	cholesterol and triglycerides	
IV	VLDL (pre-β)	triglycerides	cholesterol
V	VLDL (pre-β) and chylomicrons	triglycerides	cholesterol

Fig. 16 Lipoprotein phenotypes: lipoprotein and lipid elevations.

Apoproteins

Structural apoproteins

Lipoproteins cannot be synthesized and secreted from liver or intestine without the corresponding structural apoprotein. In addition to their structural role, apoproteins play a dynamic role in lipoprotein metabolism as enzyme activators and receptor ligands.

STRUCTURAL APOPROTEINS		
structural apoprotein	**lipoprotein**	**source**
A-I	HDL	liver intestine
B-100	VLDL, IDL, LDL	liver
B-48	chylomicrons	intestine

Fig. 17 Structural apoproteins.

ENZYME ACTIVATORS		
apoprotein	**lipoprotein**	**enzyme**
A-I	HDL3, nascent HDL	lecithin cholesterol acyl transferase
C-II	chylomicrons VLDL	lipoprotein lipase

Fig. 18 Apoproteins as enzyme activators.

Receptor ligands

apo B-100 is the binding ligand for the LDL or B,E receptor. It is synthesized in the liver, has a molecular weight of 550,000 and contains 4536 amino acid residues.

apo B-48 (mol. wt = 264,000) contains only residues 1 to 2152 (48% of apo B-100) and therefore cannot bind to the LDL receptor. It is synthesized in the intestine from the same apo B-100 gene by insertion of a stop codon into m RNA and is found only in chylomicrons and chylomicron remnants.

apo E is the binding ligand for the chylomicron remnant receptor or apo E receptor situated on the liver. It exhibits genetic polymorphism and occurs as three main isoforms (E-2, E-3, E-4) determined by three allelic genes. The affinity of apo E-2 for apo E receptors on the liver is low; apo E-2 homozygosity is associated with hyperlipidaemia and premature coronary and peripheral atherosclerosis.

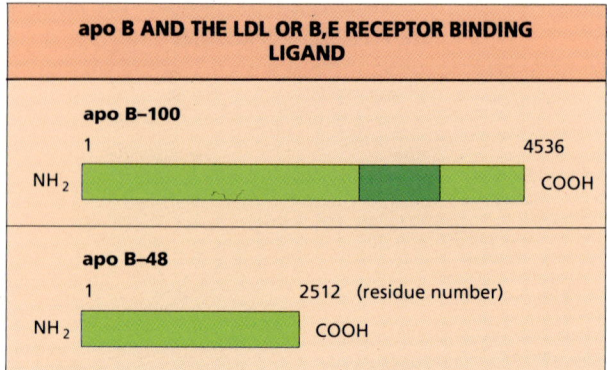

apo B AND THE LDL OR B,E RECEPTOR BINDING LIGAND

apo B–100

1   4536

NH₂   COOH

apo B–48

1   2512   (residue number)

NH₂   COOH

Fig. 19   The receptor-binding region on apo B-100 is not present on apo B-48.

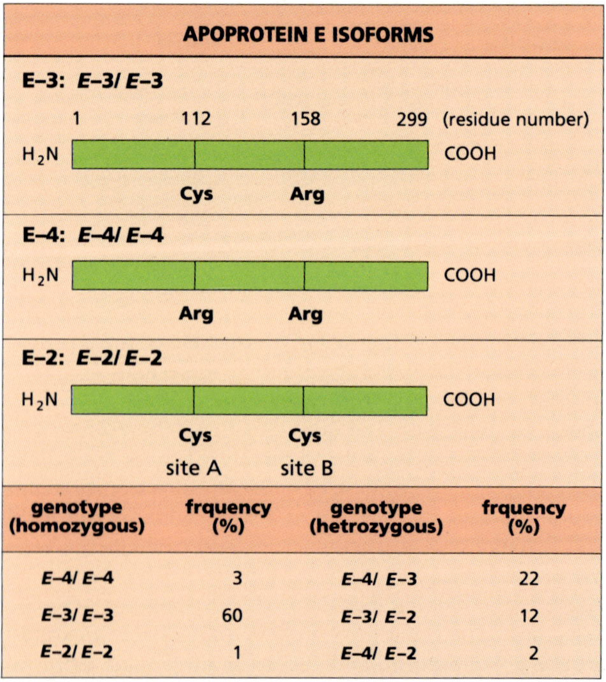

APOPROTEIN E ISOFORMS

E–3: *E–3/ E–3*

1   112   158   299   (residue number)

H₂N   COOH

            Cys   Arg

E–4: *E–4/ E–4*

H₂N   COOH

            Arg   Arg

E–2: *E–2/ E–2*

H₂N   COOH

            Cys   Cys
            site A   site B

genotype (homozygous)	frquency (%)	genotype (hetrozygous)	frquency (%)
E–4/ E–4	3	*E–4/ E–3*	22
E–3/ E–3	60	*E–3/ E–2*	12
E–2/ E–2	1	*E–4/ E–2*	2

Fig. 20   Apoproteins E isoforms and their frequencies. The isoforms differ in the amino acid substitutions at two positions in the molecule (sites A and B). Six genotypes are possible—three homozygous and three heterozygous.

THE KEY ELEMENTS OF LIPID AND LIPOPROTEIN METABOLISM

Intracellular enzymes of cholesterol metabolism and the enterohepatic circulation

Most of the cholesterol present in tissues is synthesized *de novo* rather than absorbed from the diet. Although cholesterol is produced in many tissues, the liver is the main site of synthesis in man.

Cholesterol is derived from acetate. The rate-limiting step in the sequence is catalysed by β-hydroxy-β-methylglutaryl coenzyme A (HMG CoA); synthesis of this enzyme is suppressed by cholesterol—the end product.

Bile acids are the major metabolites of cholesterol and are synthesized exclusively in the liver (300–500 mg daily). Cholesterol 7-α-hydroxylase is the rate-limiting enzyme in this process; synthesis of this enzyme is also suppressed by the end product—bile acids.

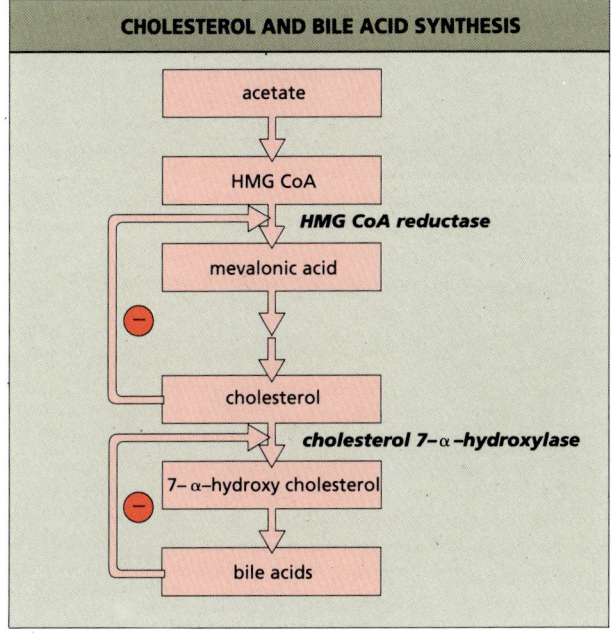

Fig. 21 Synthesis of cholesterol and bile acids.

The enterohepatic circulation

Cholesterol and bile acids are secreted into the bile and hence into the intestine. Approximately 50% of the cholesterol and 97% of the bile acids are reabsorbed and return to the liver in the portal circulation.

The secretion and reabsorption of cholesterol is dependent on its solubilization by micellar association with bile acids. Cholesterol and bile acids thus cycle continuously between the intestine and the liver with a net loss in the faeces. This enterohepatic circulation provides:

● A route for cholesterol excretion.
● Homeostatic control over hepatocyte cholesterol and bile acid concentrations by feedback regulation of HMG CoA reductase and cholesterol 7-α-hydroxylase, respectively.

Any interruption of the intestinal reabsorption of bile acids will result in increased excretion of cholesterol, both directly and by increased conversion to bile acid in the hepatocyte.

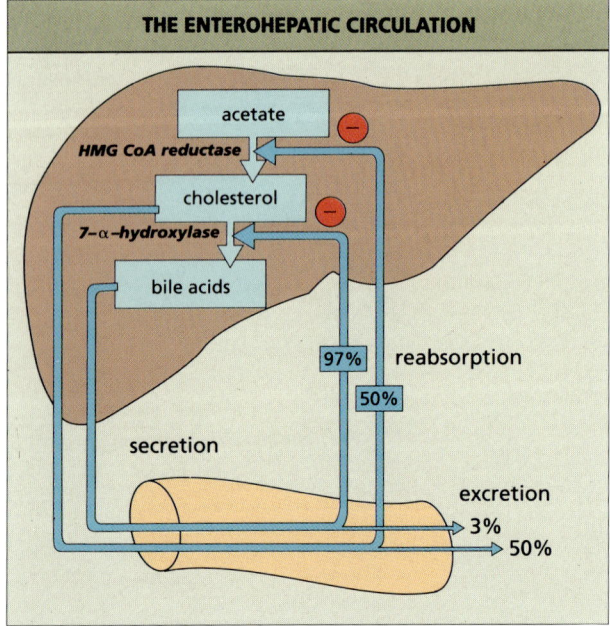

Fig. 22 The enterohepatic circulation of cholesterol and bile acids.

Fatty acid mobilization and transport

Fatty acids circulate in plasma bound to albumin. They are derived from the action of two different lipases, lipoprotein lipase and adipose tissue mobilizing enzyme.

Lipoprotein lipase (LPL) is an extracellular lipase attached by heparin sulphate to the endothelial lining of capillaries perfusing muscle and adipose tissue. It requires apo C-II as a cofactor and hydrolyses the triglyceride in triglyceride-rich lipoproteins circulating in the blood. Fatty acids can thus be released from dietary or endogenous lipoproteins and delivered to adipose tissue for storage or to muscle and liver for their metabolic requirements.

Adipose tissue mobilizing lipase (ATML), an intracellular enzyme, hydrolyses adipose tissue stores of triglyceride. It is the major source of free fatty acids (FFA) for fuel in the fasting state.

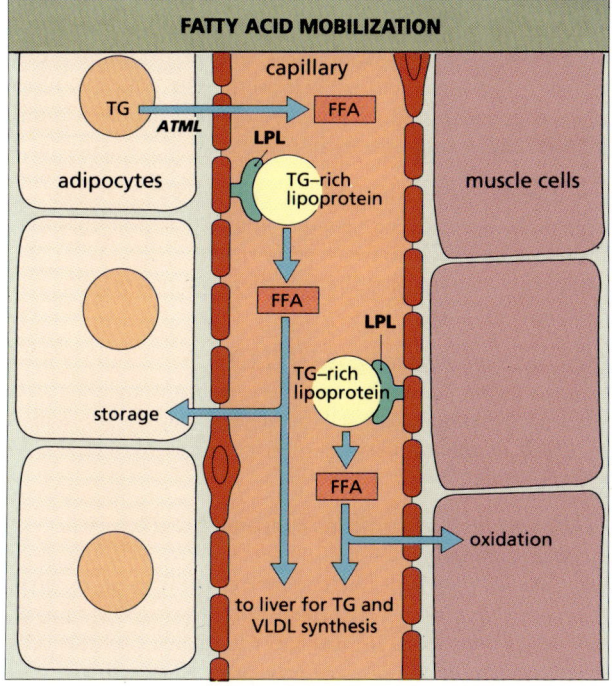

Fig. 23 Fatty acid mobilization from triglyceride in lipoproteins and adipose tissue.

Plasma enzymes, transfer proteins and reverse cholesterol transport

Lipoprotein lipase (LPL)

When triglyceride is removed from the core of chylomicrons and VLDL by the activity of LPL, the particles reduce in size and surface components (which are lamellar complexes and unesterified cholesterol, phospholipid and apo A and C) leave the particle to join the HDL pool. These are termed *surface remnants* and are considered to be an important source of HDL precursors.

Similar nascent HDL particles are secreted directly by the liver and intestine. These particles are good acceptors of unesterified cholesterol from the surface membranes of extra-hepatic cells.

Lecithin cholesterol acyl transferase (LCAT)

LCAT is synthesized in the liver and circulates in plasma. The enzyme requires apo A-I and esterifies the free cholesterol acquired by nascent HDL and HDL3 particles by transfer of a fatty acid from lecithin. The esterified cholesterol is transferred to the core of the particle forming mature, cholesterol ester-rich HDL2.

Cholesterol ester transfer protein (CETP)

This protein transfers a proportion of the cholesterol esters from mature HDL2 to triglyceride-rich lipoproteins. Triglyceride is transferred simultaneously in the reverse direction to modify HDL2.

Hepatic triglyceride lipase (HTGL)

Hepatic lipase is a similar enzyme to lipoprotein lipase. It is situated on endothelial cells in hepatic capillaries, and is involved in the conversion of triglyceride-rich HDL2 to HDL3.

HDL and reverse cholesterol transport from extra-hepatic tissues

The process by which free cholesterol is taken up by HDL from peripheral tissues, esterified and transferred to triglyceride-rich lipoproteins for transport to the liver for disposal, is termed reverse cholesterol transport. This pathway may account for the protective role of HDL against cardiovascular disease.

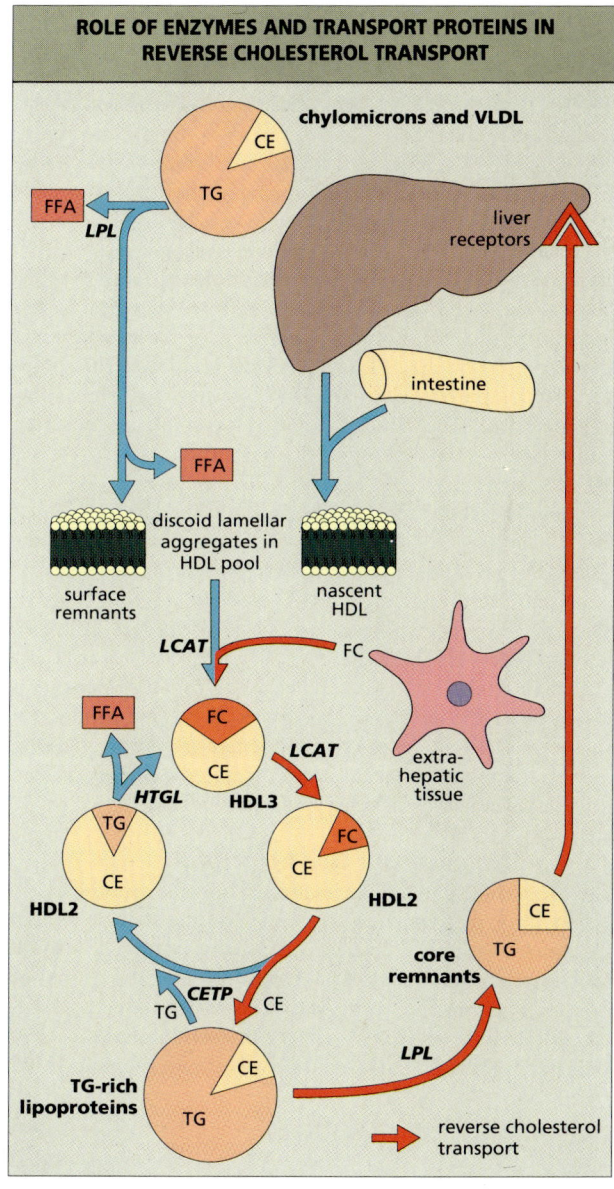

Fig. 24 Plasma enzymes, transfer proteins and reverse cholesterol transport.

Receptors

LDL receptor (B,E-receptor)

The LDL receptor binds lipoproteins containing apo B-100 and/or apo E (and hence is referred to as the B,E receptor), and will therefore bind LDL and VLDL remnants (IDL). The role of the LDL receptor is to provide cholesterol to cells throughout the body and deliver excess cholesterol to the liver for recycling or excretion as bile acids.

The receptors are synthesized in response to a fall in cellular free cholesterol concentration. Following synthesis and incorporation in the plasma membrane, the receptors cluster in coated pits on the cell surface. After binding to the receptor, an LDL particle is internalized and then undergoes lysosomal hydrolysis. The resulting increase in intracellular free cholesterol activates three regulatory mechanisms:

- The synthesis of HMG CoA reductase is suppressed—cholesterol synthesis is inhibited.
- The activity of acyl CoA:cholesterol acyltransferase (ACAT) is augmented—excess cholesterol can be stored as cholesterol esters.
- LDL receptor synthesis is inhibited—further influx of cholesterol is inhibited.

Approximately 75% of LDL cleared from the plasma is removed by the liver and 25% by extra-hepatic tissues. Of this total, 70% is cleared by LDL receptors. The remaining 30% is taken up by non-receptor mediated pathways which are not regulated by cellular cholesterol levels.

Chylomicron remnant (apo E) receptor

Chylomicron remnants are rapidly removed from the circulation by a receptor-mediated process in the liver, which recognizes the apo E on their surface but not the apo B-48. VLDL remnants that contain apo B-100 and apo E are not bound. The apo E receptor is not down-regulated by cholesterol feeding, although delivery of dietary cholesterol to the liver through this route will down-regulate LDL receptors.

HDL receptors

HDL receptors have been identified which, in contrast to LDL receptors, are up-regulated by cholesterol loading and which enable HDL3 to bind reversibly to extra-hepatic tissues, with a net efflux of cholesterol from the cell. There is also evidence for HDL receptors on the liver, which bind apo A-I and are up-regulated by cholesterol loading.

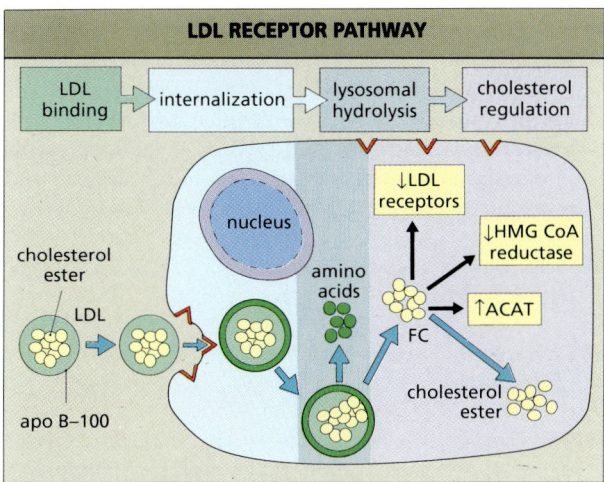

Fig. 25 The LDL receptor pathway. Adapted from Brown & Goldstein[3].

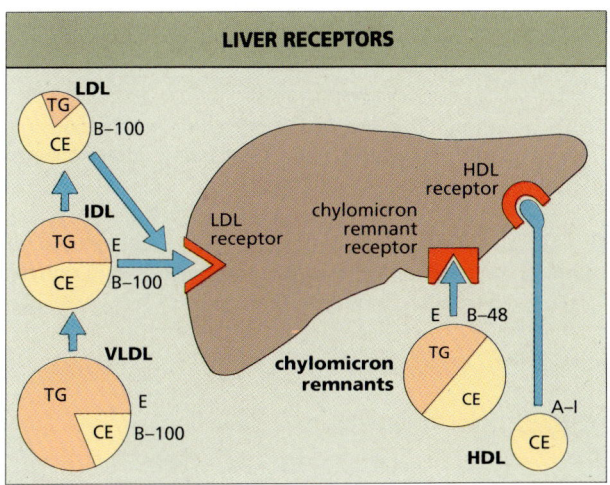

Fig. 26 Liver receptors: the chylomicron remnant, LDL and HDL receptors.

Lipoproteins and the plasma lipid transport system

Exogenous transport in chylomicrons from the intestine

● After intestinal absorption cholesterol and fatty acids from dietary fat are re-esterified to form triglycerides and cholesterol esters in intestinal mucosal cells. These lipids are then packaged together with apo B-48, phospholipid, unesterified cholesterol and several A apolipoproteins into nascent chylomicrons, secreted into the lacteals and transported via the thoracic duct into the blood.

● In the blood the chylomicrons acquire C and E apoproteins from HDL.

● Lipoprotein lipase rapidly hydrolyses the core triglyceride.

● The chylomicron reduces in size and surface remnants (lamellar complexes of free cholesterol, phospholipid, A and C apoproteins) leave the particle to join the HDL pool.

● Cholesterol ester is transferred from mature HDL to the particles in exchange for triglyceride by cholester ester transfer protein (CETP).

● The resulting core remnant, depleted of triglyceride and enriched in cholesterol ester, is of intermediate density and contains apo B-48 and apo E.

● The apo E, on the surface of the particle, is recognized by apo E receptors on hepatic parenchymal cells and rapidly removed from the blood stream.

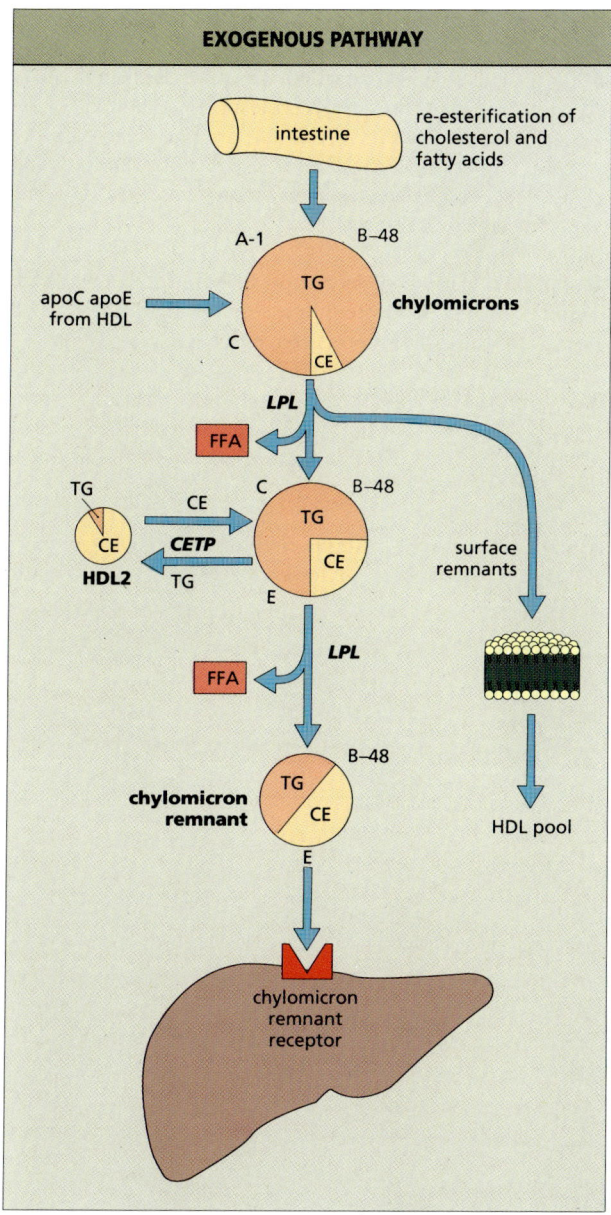

Fig. 27 The exogenous pathway of lipid transport.

Endogenous transport in VLDL from the liver

● Fatty acids surplus to oxidative requirements in the liver are esterified to form triglyceride and, in a manner analagous to chylomicron formation, are packaged together with cholesterol, cholesterol ester, phospholipid apo B-100, C apoproteins and apo E into nascent VLDL, and secreted into the blood.

● After acquisition of more apo C from HDL the VLDL interact with lipoprotein lipase and exchange lipid with HDL to form cholesterol ester-rich IDL.

● In contrast to chylomicron remnants, VLDL remnants can either be taken up by LDL receptors on the liver or undergo further delipidation by hepatic lipase, and loss of apo E, to form LDL.

● LDL are removed from the circulation by LDL receptors on the liver and, to a lesser extent, on extra-hepatic tissues.

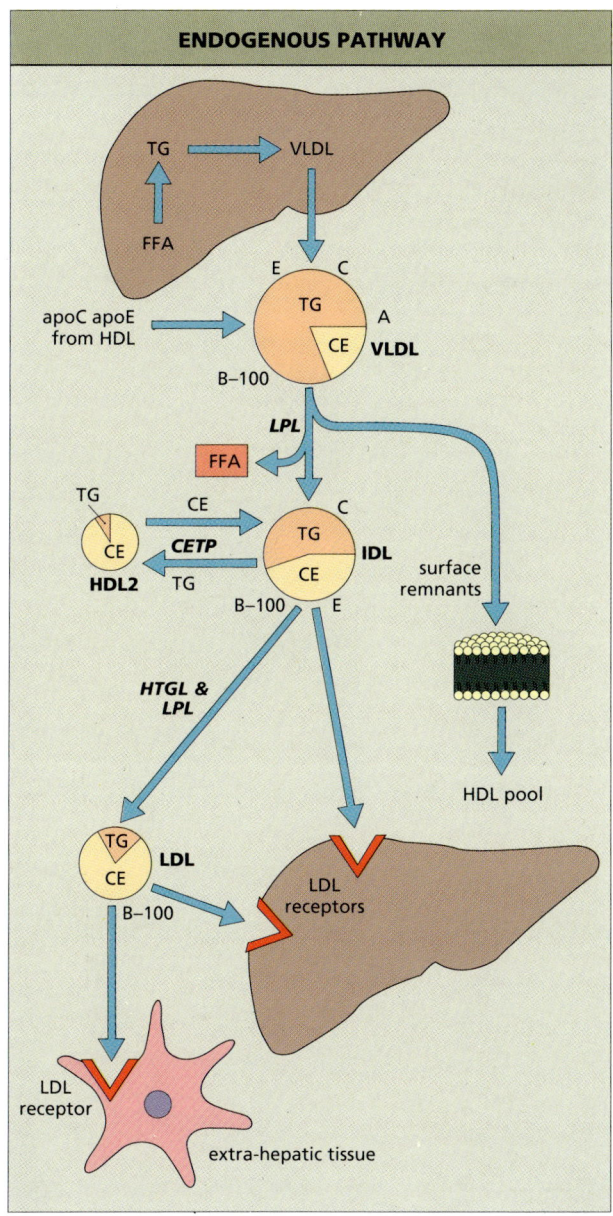

Fig. 28 The endogenous pathway of lipid transport.

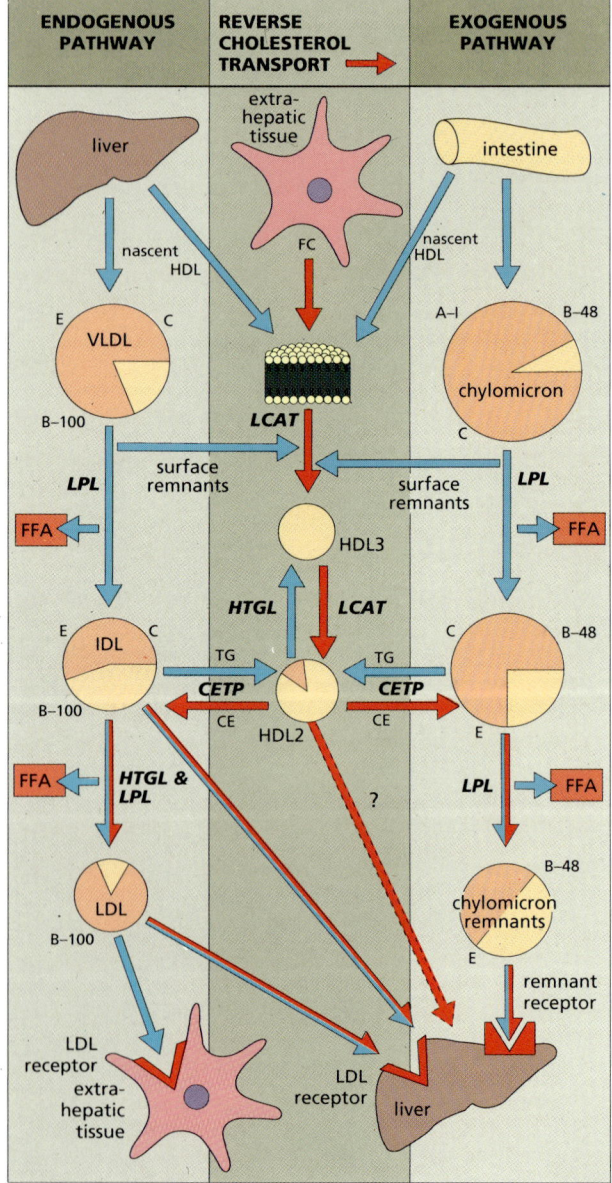

Fig. 29 An overview of exogenous and endogenous lipid transport and the role of HDL in reverse cholesterol transport.

MODE OF ACTION OF LIPID REGULATING THERAPY

Influence of diet

Cholesterol
Dietary cholesterol delivered to the liver in chylomicron remnants down-regulates LDL receptors and therefore can reduce LDL uptake and elevate cholesterol levels.

Fat
Saturated fat can be a strong factor in elevating plasma cholesterol levels. The mechanism is unclear but appears to be mediated through down-regulation of hepatic LDL receptors.

Monounsaturated and polyunsaturated fat reduce LDL and total cholesterol.

Calories
Calorie excess leads to obesity, increased fasting triglyceride levels and reduced HDL concentrations. This results from increased VLDL production and impaired catabolism of triglyceride-rich lipoproteins, which may be due to the development of insulin resistance in obese individuals.

Reduction of cholesterol intake and the proportion of calories consumed as saturated fat will reduce cholesterol levels.

Weight loss and a calorie-controlled diet will reduce triglyceride levels and elevate HDL concentration.

Mechanism of action of lipid-lowering drugs

Reduction of plasma LDL
Plasma LDL is reduced by increasing the number of LDL receptors on hepatocytes. This is achieved by reducing hepatocyte cholesterol levels and can be achieved by two mechanisms:
(1) Increasing bile acid synthesis and secretion.
(2) Inhibition of endogenous cholesterol synthesis.
Bile acid binding sequestrants (insoluble anion exchange resins) act by binding bile acids within the intestinal lumen.
HMG CoA reductase inhibitors, potent inhibitors of cholesterol synthesis especially in the liver, act by competitively

inhibiting HMG CoA reductase (the key enzyme in cellular cholesterol synthesis).

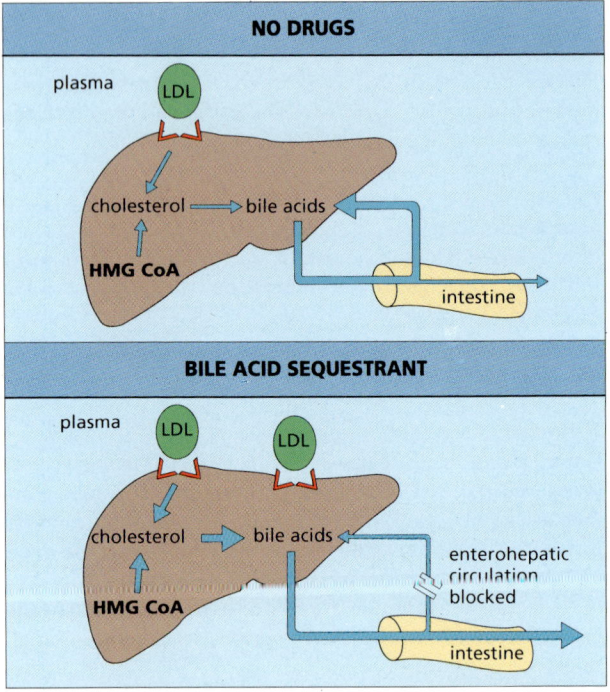

Fig. 30 Bile acid sequestrants interrupt enterohepatic circulation of bile acids. This leads to increased faecal secretion of bile acids and cholesterol and increased synthesis of bile acids in the hepatocyte. The increased requirement for cholesterol leads to up-regulation of LDL receptors in the liver and increased removal of LDL from the blood, with reduction of cholesterol levels. There is a compensatory increase in HMG CoA reductase activity and hepatocyte cholesterol synthesis which reduces the efficacy of this mechanism.

The mechanism of action of bile acid sequestrants and HMG CoA reductase inhibitors are complementary and consequently potent when used in combination. They are ineffective however in homozygous familial hypercholesterolaemia, due to the complete absence of effective LDL receptors.

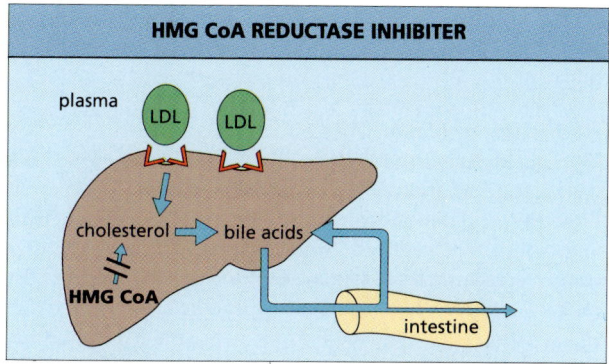

Fig. 31 HMG CoA reductase inhibitors act by competitively inhibiting HMG CoA reductase, consequently reducing cellular cholesterol levels. This leads to up-regulation of LDL receptor synthesis and increased removal of LDL from the blood, reducing blood cholesterol levels.

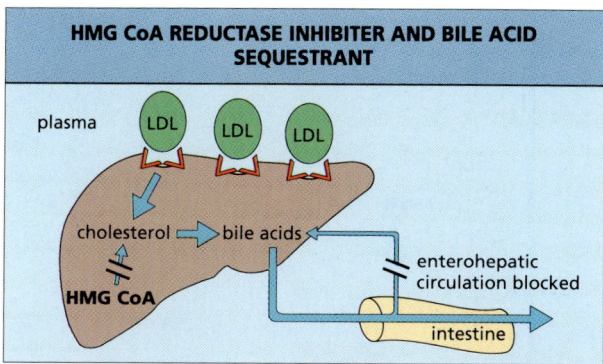

Fig. 32 Bile acid sequestrants and HMG CoA reductase inhibitors have complementary mechanisms of action, with enhanced expression of the LDL receptor.

Bile acid binding resins can elevate triglyceride and are therefore not indicated in mixed hyperlipidaemis.

Fibric acid derivative drugs also have the ability to increase LDL receptor activity. Their major effect, however, is on lowering VLDL.

Probucol reduces both LDL and HDL, but despite the latter it has been shown to cause regression of xanthelasma. There is evidence that the anti-oxidant properties of this drug prevent lipid peroxidation and hence inhibit LDL uptake by macrophages.

Reduction of plasma VLDL

Fibric acid derivatives reduce VLDL and hence triglyceride levels by stimulation of lipoprotein lipase activity.

Nicotinic acid and derivatives inhibit fatty acid release from adipocytes. The reduced influx of fatty acids into the liver suppresses synthesis of triglyceride and secretion of VLDL.

Fish oils inhibit VLDL synthesis and secretion.

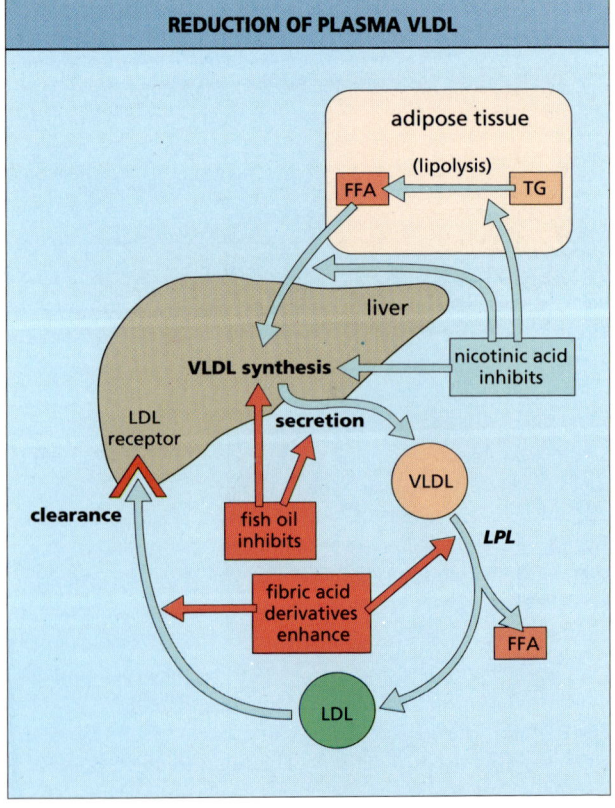

Fig. 33 Reduction of plasma VLDL by, fibric acid derivatives, nicotinic acid and derivatives, and fish oils.

HMG CoA reductase inhibitors also have a small effect on lowering production of VLDL.

MECHANISM OF ACTION OF LIPID-REGULATING THERAPY	
	mechanism of action
diet	
reduce: cholesterol / saturated fat	promotes receptor-mediated uptake of LDL
calorie reduction	decreases synthesis of VLDL
drug	
bile acid sequestrants	block bile acid reabsorption / activate cholesterol oxidation to bile acids / promote receptor-mediated uptake of LDL
HMG CoA reductase inhibitors	inhibits action of HMG CoA reductase, leading to enhanced receptor-mediated uptake of LDL
fibric acid derivatives	activate LPL and inhibit HMG CoA reductase, to increase VLDL catabolism and receptor-mediated uptake of LDL
probucol	antioxidant effect on LDL / promotes non-receptor-mediated uptake of LDL / decreases synthesis of HDL
nicotinic acid and derivatives	inhibit fatty acid release from adipocytes / inhibit VLDL synthesis and secretion
fish oils	inhibit VLDL synthesis and secretion

Fig. 34 Lipid-lowering drugs: mechanism of action.

PRIMARY DISORDERS OF LIPID METABOLISM

Primary hyperlipidaemias are genetically determined. The site of the defect has been identified in a number of disorders

PRIMARY HYPERLIPIDAEMIAS		
defect	**site**	**disorder**
enzyme	lipoprotein lipase	lipoprotein lipase deficiency
receptor	B,E receptor	familial hypercholesterolaemia
apoprotein	apo E	apo E-2 homozygosity (remnant hyperlipidaemia)
	apo C-II	Apo C-II deficiency
defect uncertain		hyperalphalipo-proteinaemia
		familial hypertriglyceridaemia
		familial combined hyperlipidaemia
		polygenic hypercholesterolaemia

Fig. 35 Primary hyperlipidaemias.

but in some of the most common it remains uncertain. The frequently occurring hyperlipidaemias result from a combination of genetic and environmental factors (for example, polygenic hypercholesterolaemia).

lipoprotein abnormality	major lipid elevation
chylomicrons	triglyceride
LDL	cholesterol
IDL	cholesterol, triglyceride
chylomicrons	triglyceride
HDL	cholesterol
VLDL (rarely chylomicrons)	triglyceride
LDL, VLDL	cholesterol triglyceride
LDL	cholesterol

PRIMARY HYPERLIPIDAEMIAS: PREVALENCE AND CLINICAL FEATURES		
disorder	prevalence	transmission
lipoprotein lipase deficiency	very rare	autosomal recessive
familial hypercholesterolaemia		autosomal dominant
homozygote	1:1,000,000	
heterozygote	1:500	
apo E2 homozygosity	1:10,000	polygenic
apo C-II deficiency	very rare	autosomal recessive
hyperalphalipo-proteinaemia	varies	polygenic
familial hypertriglyceridaemia	1:600	autosomal dominant
familial combined hyperlipidaemia	1:300	? polygenic ? autosomal dominant
polygenic hypercholesterolaemia	common	polygenic

Fig. 36 Prevalence and clinical features of the primary hyperlipidaemias. Of the most common primary hyperlipidaemias familial combined hyperlipidaemia polygenic hypercholesterolaemia

clinical features		
clinical signs	pancreatitis risk	atherosclerosis risk
hepatosplenomegaly eruptive xanthomas lipaemia retinalis	+	−
corneal arcus xanthelasmas tendonous xanthomas		
tuberous xanthomas	−	+++
	−	++
palmar crease xanthomas tuberous xanthomas tubero-eruptive xanthoma	−	++
hepatosplenomegaly eruptive xanthomas lipaemia retinalis	+	−
	−	−

in severe forms:
  hepatosplenomegaly
  eruptive xanthomas
  lipaemia retinalis
	+	?+

corneal arcus xanthelasmas	−	++
corneal arcus xanthelasmas	−	+

and familial hypertriglyceridaemia are seen in adulthood and often occur in the absence of clinical signs. In familial combined hyperlipidaemia the lipoprotein phenotype varies within families.

Familial hypercholesterolaemia (FH)

This condition is characterized by a raised plasma total and LDL-cholesterol. It is due to impaired LDL receptor activity resulting from either a reduction in the synthesis of LDL receptors or the production of defective LDL receptors; 'receptor-negative' patients have a worse clinical outcome.

The homozygous condition is characterized by the absence of effective LDL receptor activity. The heterozygous condition (the commonest single-gene disorder in clinical practice) has 50% of the normal number of LDL receptors. There is commonly a family history of premature coronary heart disease (CHD) in first degree relatives occurring at ages <50 years or in secondary relatives <60 years.

FAMILIAL HYPERCHOLESTEROLAEMIA		
	homozygote	**heterozygote**
cholesterol	usually >15.5 mmol/l 600 mg/dl	usually >7.8 mmol/l 300 mg/dl
clinical features: cutaneous	tendon xanthoma tuberous xanthomas	tendon xanthoma xanthelasma
corneal arcus	corneal arcus may be seen before 20 years	common
polyarthritis	during adolescence	uncommon
premature atherosclerosis	CHD often within 2nd decade aortic ejection murmur (from aortic root atheroma)	CHD within 4–5th decade

Fig. 37   Characteristics of familial hypercholesterolaemia.

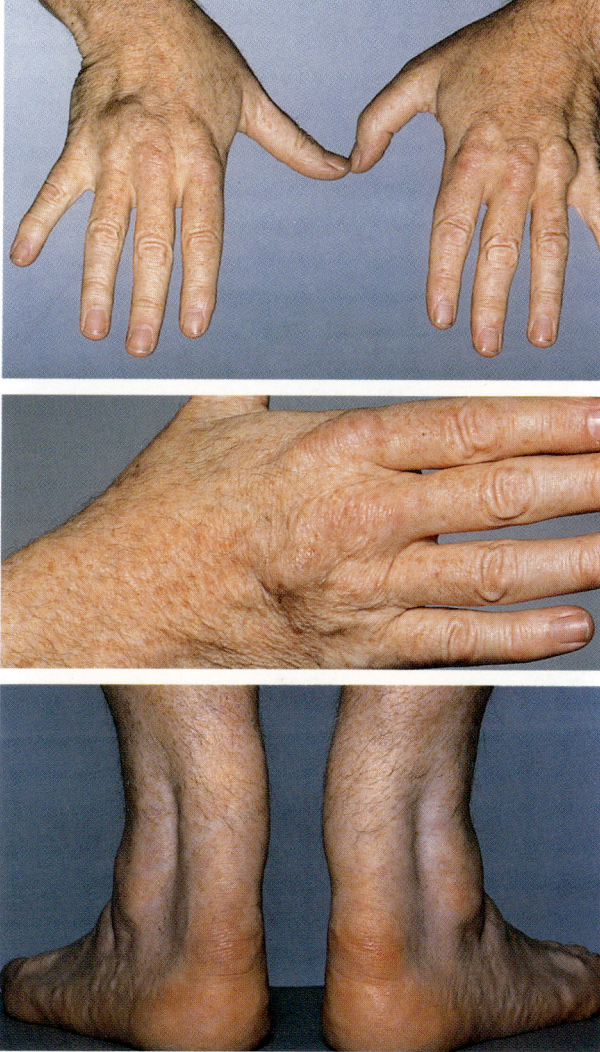

Fig. 38 Xanthomas are a pathological deposition of lipid in skin and tissues due to both the severity and the duration of hypercholesterolaemia. Tendon xanthomas strongly suggest familial hypercholesterolaemia and may occur in the extensor tendons of the hands (upper, middle), the achilles tendon (lower), and insertion of the patella tendon.

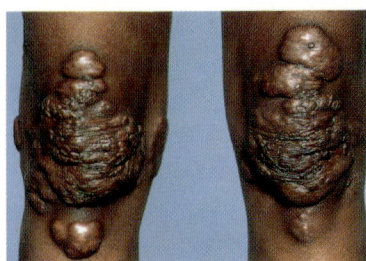

Fig. 39 Planar or tuberous xanthomas may be seen in homozygous familial hypercholesterolaemia and in apo E-2 homozygosity.

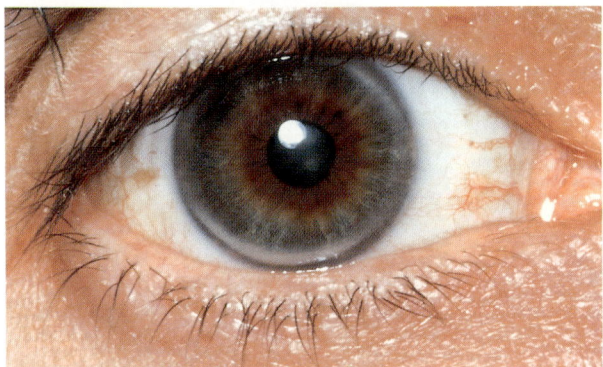

Fig. 40 Corneal arcus commonly occurs in familial hypercholesterolaemia and other causes of hypercholesterolaemia, as well as in older people with normal lipids.

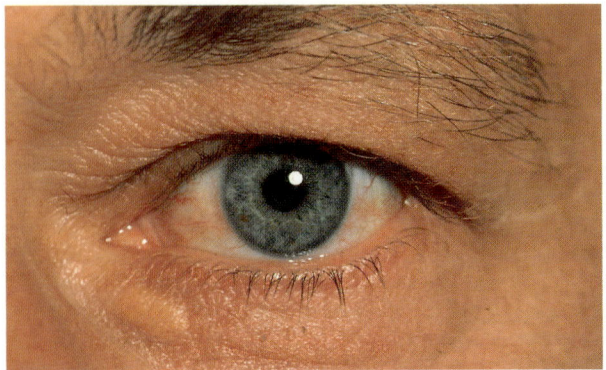

Fig. 41 Eyelid xanthelasma are commonly seen in normocholesterolaemic and hypercholesterolaemic subjects.

apo E-2 homozygosity

The genotype of this condition occurs with a frequency of 1:100. A hyperlipidaemia is only expressed in 1% of these individuals when a further genetic or metabolic abnormality (for example, obesity, diabetes or hypothyroidism) exacerbates the diminished ability to clear IDL (chylomicron or VLDL remnants).

APO E-2 HOMOZYGOSITY	
cholesterol increase	usually >7.8 mmol/l >300 mg/dl
triglyceride increase	usually >5.0 mmol/l >442 mg/dl
clinical features: cutaneous	palmar crease (orange-coloured) xanthomas tuberous and tuberoeruptive xanthomas
premature atherosclerosis	peripheral vascular disease as well as cerebrovascular disease and CHD occur

Fig. 42 Lipid elevations and clinical features of apo E-2 homozygosity (remnant hyperlipidaemia).

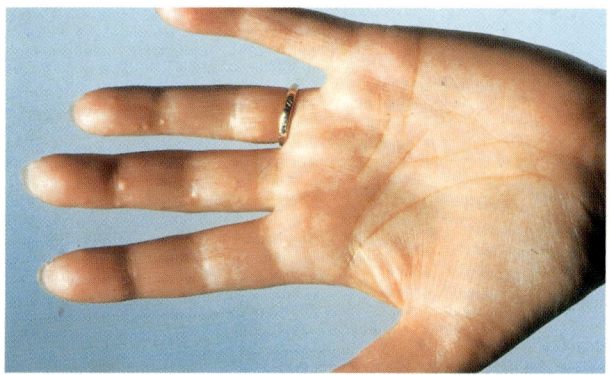

Fig. 43 Palmar crease xanthomas. .

Familial chylomicronaemia syndrome

Severe hypertriglyceridaemia of the familial chylomicronaemia syndrome, due to either lipoprotein lipase deficiency or
apoprotein C-II deficiency, is a rare childhood condition; the
clinical features include pancreatitis, hepatomegaly, lipae-
mia retinalis and eruptive xanthomas. These clinical find-
ings are also seen in severe forms of familial
hypertriglyceridaemia.

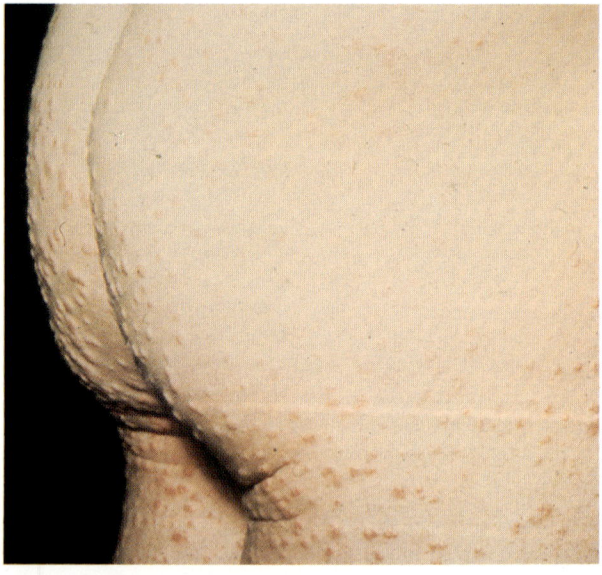

Fig. 44 Eruptive xanthomas are a feature of the familial
chylomicronaemia syndrome.

SECONDARY CAUSES OF HYPERLIPIDAEMIA

Secondary hyperlipidaemias are relatively common and may account for up to 40% of all hyperlipidaemias. The lipid abnormalities are often reversible with appropriate management of the underlying condition. Occasionally primary and secondary disorders of lipid metabolism co-exist.

CAUSES OF SECONDARY HYPERLIPIDAEMIA			
	lipid changes		
	cholesterol	triglyceride	HDL
conditions obesity	→ ↑	↑	↓
diabetes mellitus			
untreated	→ ↑	↑	↓
IDDM (treated)			→ ↑
NIDDM (treated)		↑	↓
hypothyroidism	↑		
chronic renal failure	→ ↑	↑	↓
nephrotic syndrome	↑	↑	↓
biliary obstruction	↑		
myeloma	↑	↑	
glycogen storage disease	↑		
drugs alcohol excess		↑	
thiazides	↑	↑	→ ↓
beta-blockers		↑	↓
corticosteroids		↑	
oestrogens		↑	↑
progestagens	↑	↑	↓

Fig. 45 Causes of secondary hyperlipidaemia.

Mechanisms of hyperlipidaemia in obesity and diabetes

Obesity and non-insulin dependent diabetes mellitus (NIDDM)

Increased hepatic triglyceride production and secretion of VLDL results from:

● high calorie intake
● insulin resistance promoting lipolysis in adipose tissue and increased delivery of FFA to the liver.

Decreased clearance of triglyceride-rich lipoproteins and low HDL levels result from reduced lipoprotein lipase activity in insulin resistant states

Insulin-dependent diabetes mellitus (IDDM)

Lack of insulin in uncontrolled diabetes has a similar effect on lipid metabolism to insulin resistance

Diabetes mellitus

Lipid abnormalities are associated with the development of macrovascular disease; diabetic microvascular complications may also occur in these patients

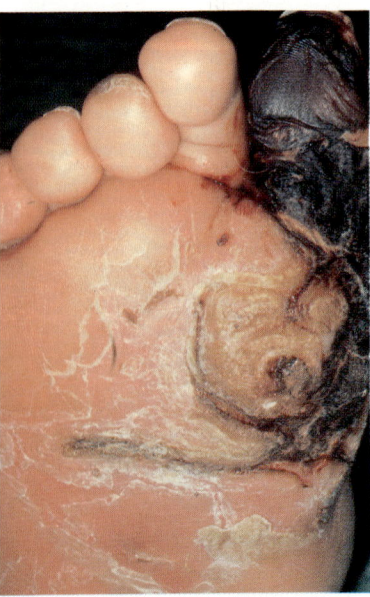

Fig.46 Diabetic gangrene due to ischaemia; lipid abnormalities may contribute to the vascular disease.

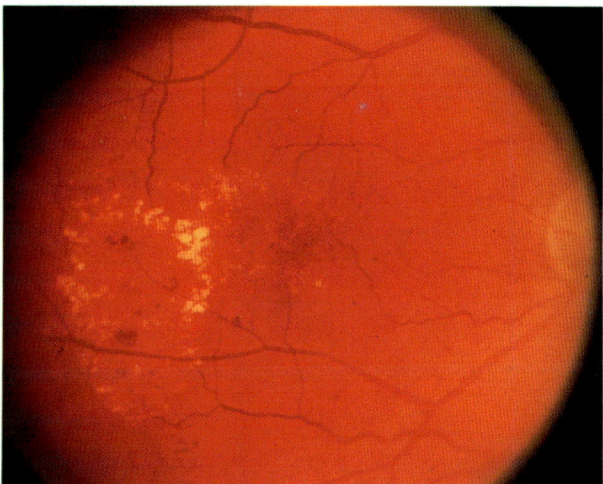

Fig. 47 Diabetic retinopathy with macular changes. This may be seen in NIDDM; lipid changes are commonly seen in these patients.

Clinical signs and mechanisms of hyperlipidaemia in other conditions

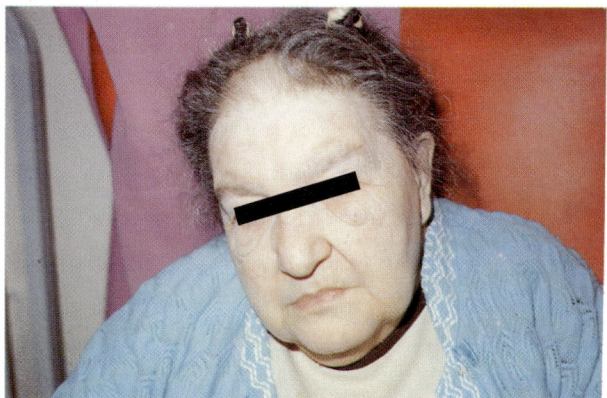

Fig. 48 Hypothyroidism: typical facies of hypothyroidism with loss of hair, periorbital swelling and puffy features.
  Hypercholesterolaemia results from decreased LDL receptor activity and reduced hepatic excretion of cholesterol as a consequence of low thyroid hormone levels.

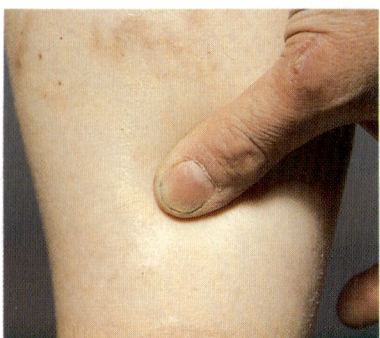
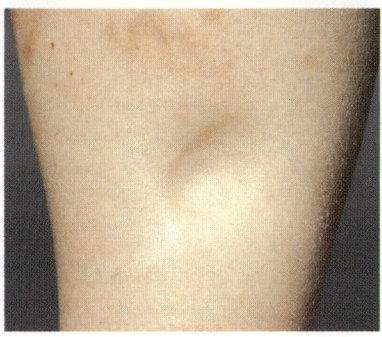

Fig. 49 Peripheral oedema of the nephrotic syndrome.

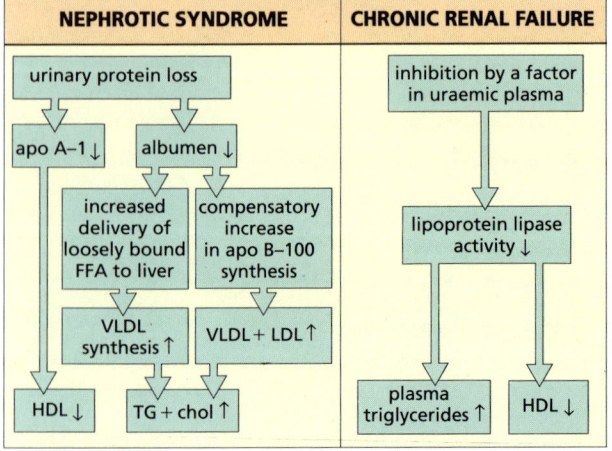

Fig. 50 Mechanisms of hyperlipidaemia in nephrotic syndrome and chronic renal failure.

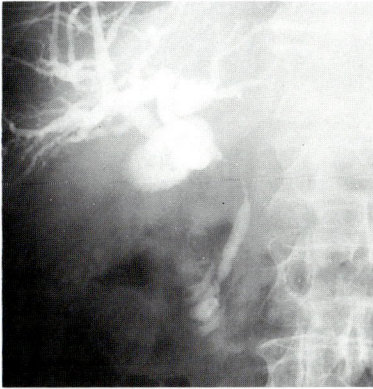

Fig. 51 Biliary obstruction (extrahepatic): cholangiogram showing stricture of the common bile duct with dilated biliary tree.

Intrahepatic or extrahepatic obstruction to the excretion of bile results in an increase in plasma cholesterol; the mechanism is not fully understood.

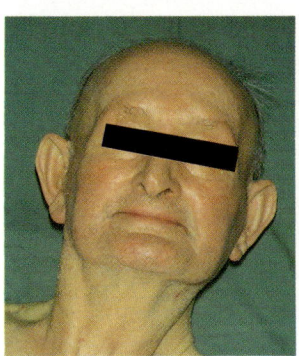 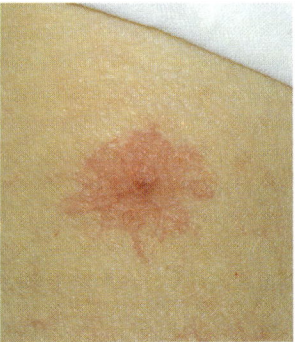

Fig. 52 Jaundice (left) and spider naevus (right) associated with chronic liver disease.

Severe liver disease results in a range of lipid abnormalities that may be associated with reduction of enzyme and receptor activities in addition to failure of excretory function.

CAUSES OF HYPERTRIGLYCERIDAEMIA OF ALCOHOL EXCESS
decreased fatty acid oxidation
preferential oxidation of ethanol in the liver
enhanced triglyceride production and VLDL secretion.

Fig. 53 Hypertriglyceridaemia of alcohol excess.

LIPIDS, LIPOPROTEINS AND VASCULAR DISEASE

Atherosclerosis

The fundamental lesion of atherosclerosis is the atheromatous or fibro-fatty plaque. Atherosclerosis develops over several years and may be asymptomatic. It tends to affect the inner walls of large and medium-sized arteries, resulting in narrowing of the vessel. Symptomatic atherosclerosis may occur in minutes and the clinical consequences can include coronary artery disease (angina pectoris, myocardial infarction, acute cardiac death), cerebrovascular disease or peripheral vascular disease (claudication, gangrene).

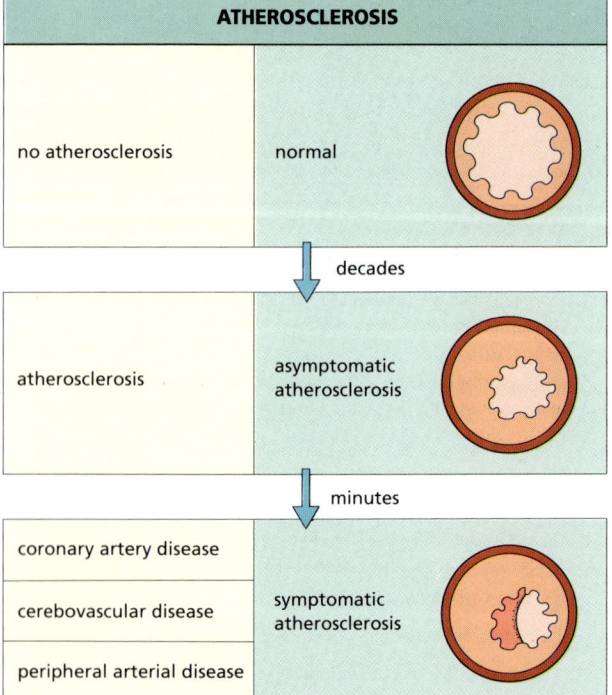

Fig. 54 The progression of atherosclerosis

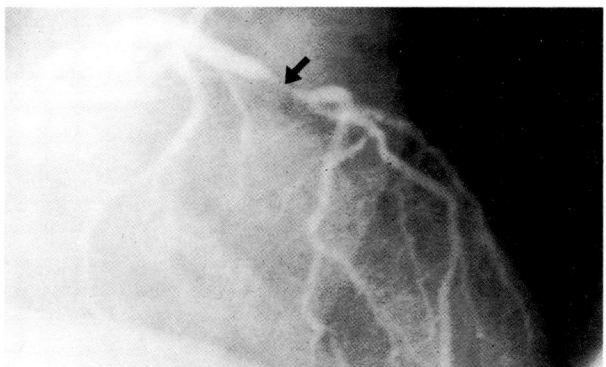

Fig. 55 Coronary artery disease. Coronary angiogram showing critical stenosis of left anterior descending coronary artery.

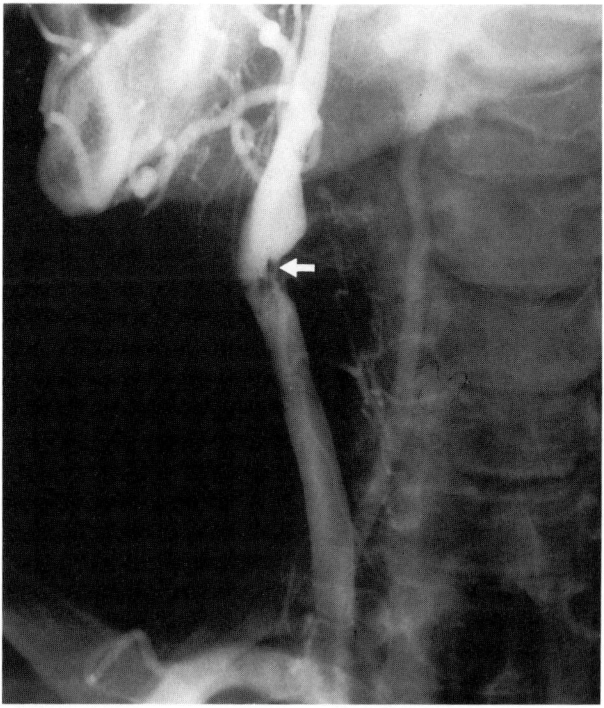

Fig. 56 Cerebrovascular disease. Carotid angiogram showing atherosclerotic narrowing of internal carotid artery.

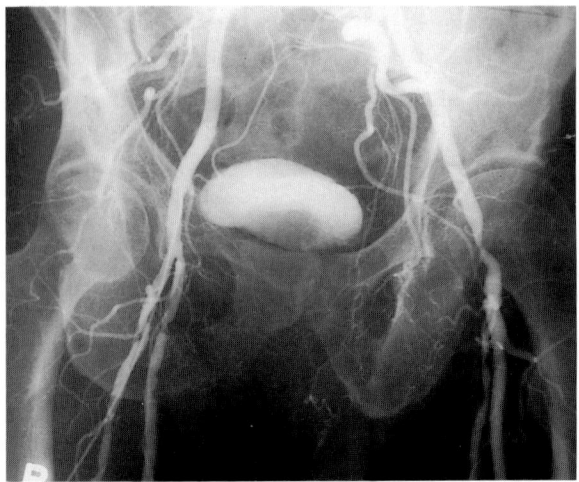

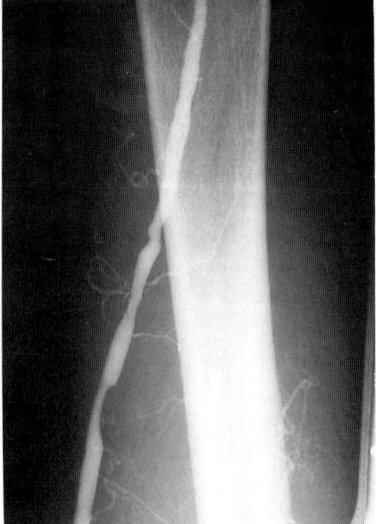

Fig. 57 Peripheral vascular disease. Arteriogram of iliofemoral (upper) and femoral (lower) arteries showing irregular narrowing due to atherosclerotic disease.

The stages of atherosclerosis

The different stages of atherosclerosis are characterized by the early lesion (or fatty streak), the advanced lesion (or fibrous plaque), and the complicated lesion with ulceration, calcification or haemorrhage. Several factors are involved in the process, including lipids, lipoproteins, platelets and clotting factors.

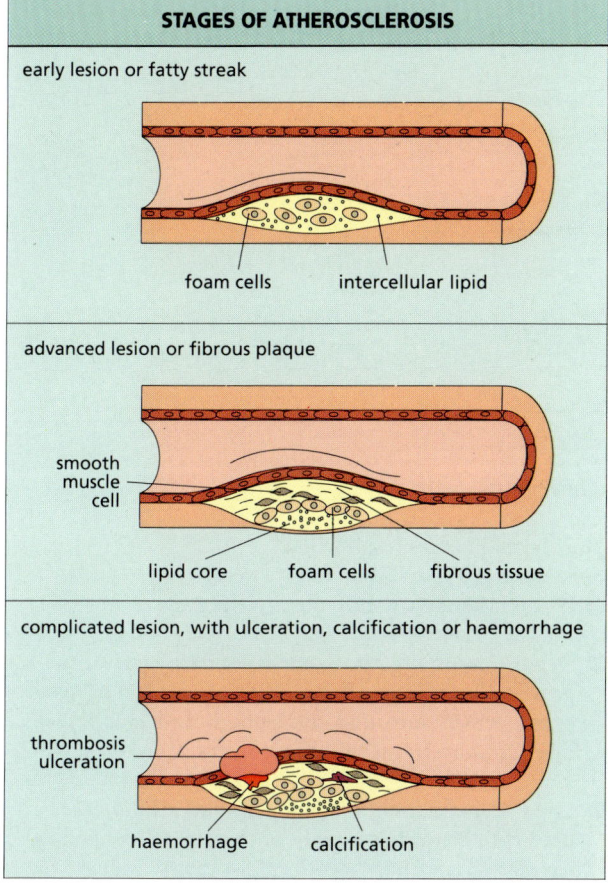

STAGES OF ATHEROSCLEROSIS

early lesion or fatty streak

foam cells   intercellular lipid

advanced lesion or fibrous plaque

smooth muscle cell

lipid core   foam cells   fibrous tissue

complicated lesion, with ulceration, calcification or haemorrhage

thrombosis ulceration

haemorrhage   calcification

Fig. 58 Stages of atherosclerosis: the fatty streak, the fibrous plaque and the complicated lesion (leading to gangrene, aneurysmal dilatation or infarction).

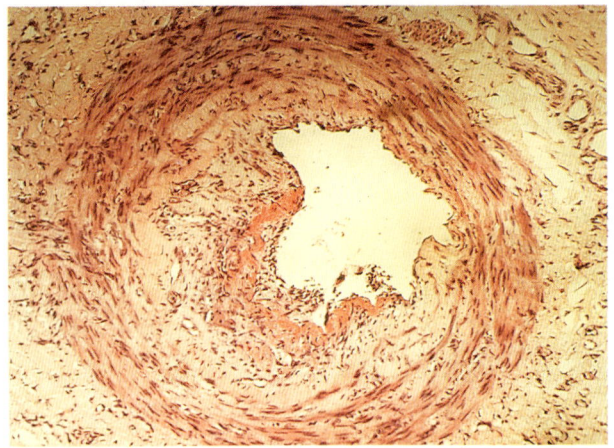

Fig. 59 Histological section of artery showing atherosclerotic narrowing of lumen.

The lesions

The fibrous plaques result from:

● Proliferation of smooth muscle cells.

● Deposition of large amounts of connective tissue matrix proteins (including collagen, elastic fibres and proteoglycans), which surround the smooth and muscle cells. Fibrous tissue forms the main constituent of the plaque.

● Lipid accumulation in foam cells and a lipid core. The lipid core comprises mainly of cholesterol derived from circulation and not from local synthesis. Macrophages (derived from monocytes) become foam cells by ingesting cholesterol from LDL. The foam cell is the distinctive feature of the atherosclerotic plaque.

The early lesion is an accumulation of lipid, macrophages and smooth muscle cells in the subendothelial area in the intima. It is not entirely clear whether all early lesions progress to the more complicated atherosclerotic lesions. Advanced lesions, or fibrous plaques, become more common with age, but they may also be seen in young individuals with some genetic forms of hyperlipidaemia. When the fibrous plaque progresses to the complicated lesion arterial flow is compromised.

Theories of atherosclerosis
As atherosclerosis is considered to be a multifactorial process, several theories have been suggested to explain atherogenesis. Many include the increased uptake of lipoproteins into the arterial wall, the accumulation of lipids in the arterial wall and transport of lipids from arterial wall as part of the process.

The 'response to injury' hypothesis; states that stimuli damage the vascular endothelium to initiate the process.

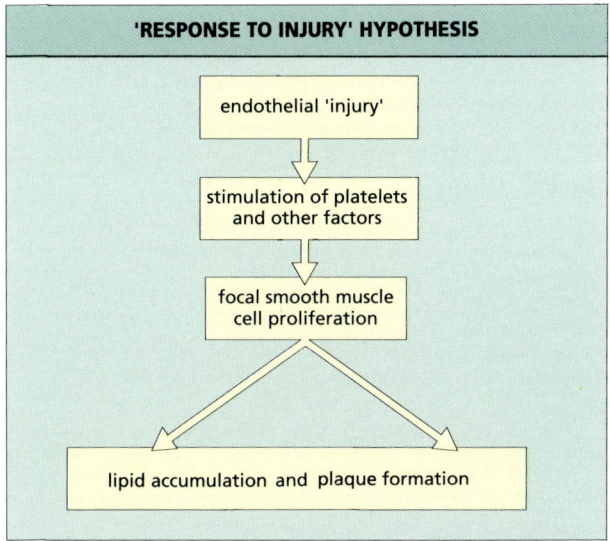

Fig. 60   The 'response to injury' hypothesis of pathogenesis of atherosclerosis.[4] The initiating stimuli may be mechanical, chemical, toxic, viral or immunological (e.g. hypertension, smoking, increased LDL).

Cholesterol and coronary heart disease (CHD)

The strong positive relationship between cholesterol and CHD comes from several lines of evidence.

CHOLESTEROL AND CHD: EVIDENCE FOR POSITIVE RELATIONSHIP		
epidemiological evidence	1. Between populations	Seven Countries study[5]
	2. Migration study	Japanese living in Japan, Hawaii and San Francisco[6]
	3. Within a single population	Multiple Risk Factor Intervention Trial[7,8] British Regional Heart Study[9]
clinical studies	several genetic hyperlipidaemias in man are associated with premature CHD	
clinical trial evidence	cholesterol-lowering by either diet or drug therapy is associated with a reduction in CHD	
experimental animal studies	cholesterol feeding in rabbits induces hypercholesterolaemiamia and premature atherosclerosis	
in vitro experimental studies	studies on the mechanisms of atherogenesis confirm a causative link with cholesterol and LDL	

Fig. 61 Evidence for a strong positive relationship between cholesterol and coronary heart disease.

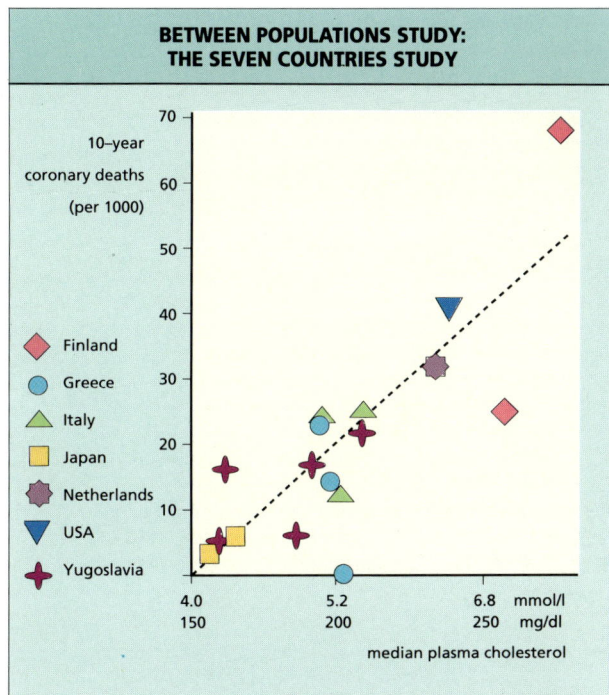

**BETWEEN POPULATIONS STUDY:
THE SEVEN COUNTRIES STUDY**

10–year coronary deaths (per 1000)

- Finland
- Greece
- Italy
- Japan
- Netherlands
- USA
- Yugoslavia

median plasma cholesterol

Fig. 62 Between populations study: the Seven Countries study.[5] In this study involving 12,763 men in 16 different regions from seven countries, the median cholesterol levels were highly correlated with CHD mortality.

MIGRATION STUDY			
	Japan	**Hawaii**	**San Francisco**
cholesterol			
mmol/l	4.7	5.6	5.9
mg/dl	181	218	228
CHD rate per 1000	25.4	34.7	44.6

Fig. 63 Migration study: cholesterol levels and CHD rates in Japanese living in Japan, Hawaii and San Francisco.[6]

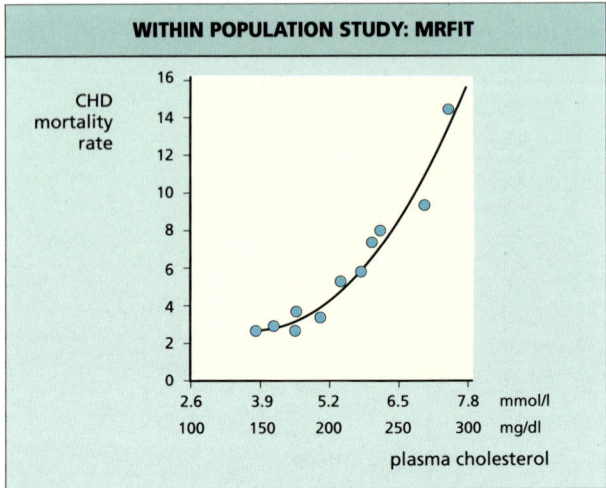

Fig. 64 Within population study: the Multiple Risk Factor Intervention Trial (MRFIT)[7,8] in the USA surveyed over 360,000 men aged 35–57. CHD mortality increased with increasing levels of cholesterol.

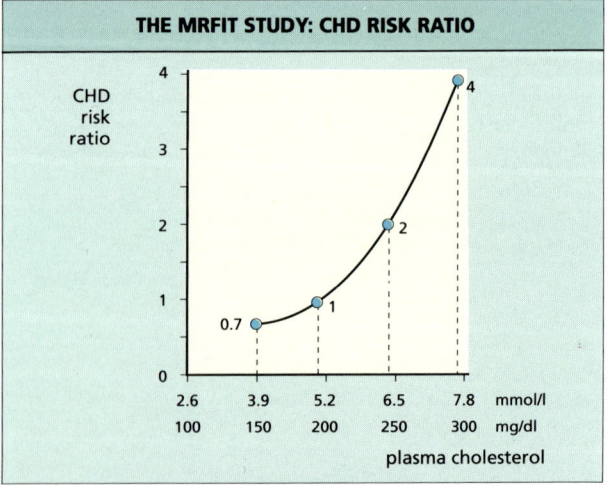

Fig. 65 The MRFIT study.[7,8] The lowest CHD rates occurred when cholesterol was 5.2 mmol/l (200 mg/dl) or below. The risk of CHD was doubled at 6.5 mmol/l (250 mg/dl) and quadrupled at 7.8 mmol/l (300 mg/dl). (Coronary mortality expressed as risk ratio).

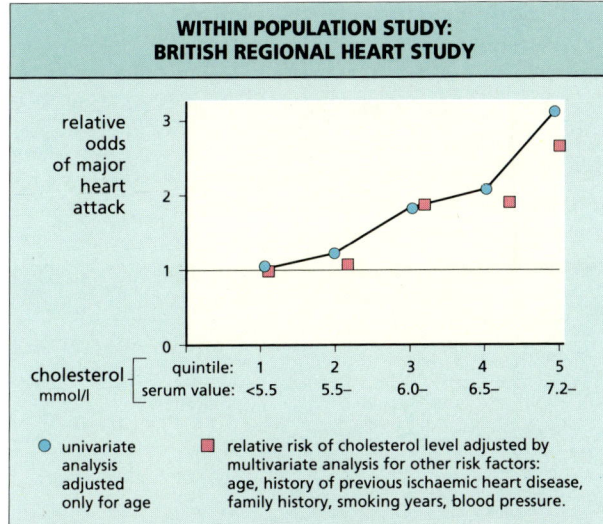

Fig. 66 Within population study: the British Regional Heart study[9] of 7735 men showed that the relationship of cholesterol to CHD was independent of other risk factors.

LDL and coronary heart disease

The association of LDL-cholesterol is stronger than that for cholesterol alone.

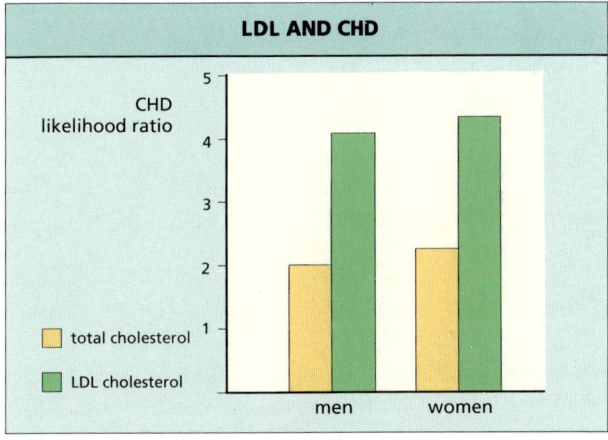

Fig. 67 Likelihood ratios for CHD with respect to total cholesterol and LDL-cholesterol in the Framingham Heart Study.

Triglyceride and coronary heart disease

The association of triglyceride levels and CHD remains controversial. However there is evidence from the Framingham Heart Study[10] that a combination of an elevated serum TG with a reduced HDL is strongly associated with CHD for men and women.

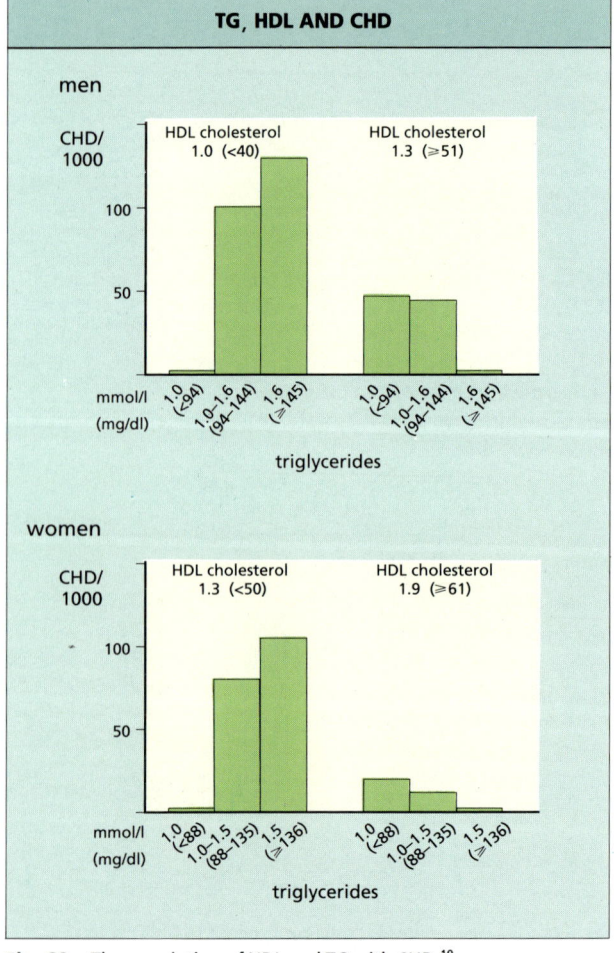

Fig. 68 The association of HDL and TG with CHD.[10]

HDL and coronary heart disease

HDL promotes the transport of extrahepatic cholesterol back to the liver for elimination. This 'reverse cholesterol transport' may explain the strong association of a reduced HDL with CHD, and a high HDL being 'cardio-protective'. The predictive power of a reduced HDL-cholesterol for CHD, independent of other risk factors, has been demonstrated in several epidemiologic studies.

STUDIES LINKING LOW HDL WITH CHD	
area/country	study
North America	Framingham[10]
	LRCF[11]
	LRC-CPPT[12]
	MRFIT[13]
Europe	PROCAM[14]
UK	British Regional Heart Study[15]
Israel	Israeli IHD study[16]
Scandinavia	Tromso[17]
	Oslo[18]

Fig. 69 Prospective epidemiological studies showing significant inverse associations of HDL-cholesterol and cardiovascular disease. The association of a reduced HDL-cholesterol and CHD is stronger than for any other single lipid or lipoprotein fraction.

Cholesterol ratios and coronary heart disease

Since the different cholesterol fractions are independently related to the risk of CHD, an assessment of risk is often expressed as the ratio of total cholesterol/HDL-cholesterol. A ratio of 4.5 is considered to have a risk ratio of 1

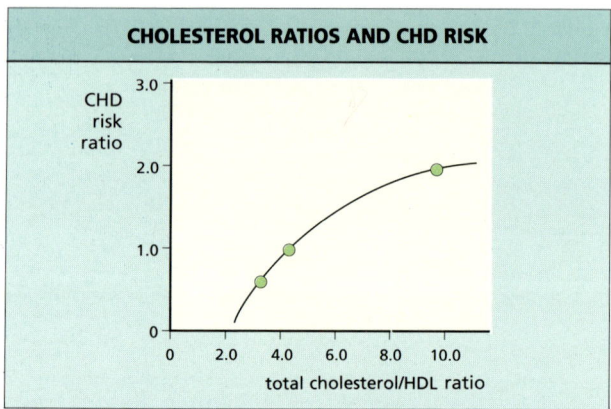

Fig. 70   Cholesterol ratios and CHD risk (Framingham Heart Study).

Apoproteins and coronary heart disease

APOPROTEINS AND CHD	
apo A and apo B	in cross-sectional studies apo A-I and apo B have been shown to be better discriminators for the presence of coronary disease than their respective lipoproteins HDL and LDL the predictive value of these apoproteins for subsequent CHD has not been established
Lp(a)	Lp(a), an LDL-like particle, containing apo B-100 and apo (a), is elevated in subjects with CHD apo (a) is structurally similar to plasminogen, indicating that this particle has a potential role in thrombogenesis as well as atherogenesis

Fig. 71   Apoproteins and CHD.

Non-lipid risk factors and coronary heart disease

These risk factors act independently and are additive when they co-exist (sometimes synergistically).

NON-LIPID RISK FACTORS FOR CHD	
modifiable	**not modifiable**
hypertension	age
smoking	gender
diabetes mellitus	family history
obesity	personality
lack of exercise	stress

Fig. 72 Non-lipid risk factors for CHD.

NON-LIPID FACTORS AND CHOLESTEROL AND CHD		
	death rate per 1000	
	low cholesterol	**high cholesterol**
non-smoker normal BP	1.6	6.4
non-smoker raised BP	3.7	10.7
smoker normal BP	5.2	13.3
smoker raised BP	6.3	21.4

Fig. 73 Relation between non-lipid risk factors and serum cholesterol (lowest 20% and highest 20% of the population) and death from CHD.[8]

CHANGES IN LIPIDS AND LIPOPROTEINS WITH ANTIHYPERTENSIVE THERAPY				
drugs	total cholesterol	LDL-C	HDL-C	TG
diuretcs	↑	↑	→ ↓	↑
β- blockers B₁ - and non-selective	→	→	↓	↑
intrinsic sympathomimetic activity	→	→	→ ↑	↑
α- blockers	↓	↓	↑	↓
vasodilators calcium antagonists ACE inhibitors	→	→	→	→

Fig. 74 Treatment of hypertension with many commonly used antihypertensive drugs has been associated with changes in lipids and lipoproteins.

Relative importance of the major risk factors for vascular disease

MAJOR RISK FACTORS AND VASCULAR DISEASE			
	coronary arteries	cerebral arteries	femoral arteries
lipids and lipoproteins	+++	−	+
hypertension	+	+++	−
smoking	++	−	+++

Fig. 75 Relative importance of the major risk factors associated with vascular disease.

WHY TREAT LIPID DISORDERS?

- **To prevent pancreatitis**, which is associated with high levels of serum triglycerides (> 11.0 mmol/l, 1000 mg/dl) and can be avoided by reduction of triglycerides to normal levels.
- **To reduce atherosclerosis**

Evidence that treating lipid disorders reduces atherosclerosis

Several clinical trials have assessed the effect of reduction of total cholesterol, elevation of HDL and triglyceride lowering on atherosclerotic disease.

The trials are of two types:

- lipid-lowering trials, with lowering as the only intervention.

- multiple risk factor intervention trials: treatment of lipid abnormalities together with modification of other risk factors.

Lipid-lowering trials
Lipid-lowering trials have assessed the effect of treatment with either diet alone or in combination with drug therapy on:

- Clinical end-points of CHD, either fatal or non-fatal myocardial infarction in individuals without (primary prevention trial) or with (secondary prevention trial) clinical evidence of coronary disease.

- Rate of progression and regression of atherosclerosis in native vessels or bypass grafts, measured angiographically.

The majority of trials have studied males of between 30 and 65 years of age.

LIPID MODIFICATION IN RELATION TO CHD	number in study	duration (years)
primary prevention trials		
LA Veterans study[19]	846	8
WHO Cooperative Trial of Clofibrate[20]	15,745	5
Lipid Research Clinics Coronary Primary Prevention Trial[21] (LRC-CPPT)	3806	7.4
Helsinki Heart Study[22]	4081	5
Secondary prevention trials Coronary Drug Project (niacin group)[23]	3908	5
Stockholm Ischaemic Heart Disease Secondary Prevention Study[24]	555	5

Fig. 76 Lipid modification in relation to CHD.

LIPID MODIFICATION WITH ANGIOGRAPHIC ASSESSMENT	number in study	duration (years)
coronary artery disease		
Finnish Regression Study[25]	28	7
NHLBI Type II Coronary Intervention Study[26]	116	5
Cholesterol-Lowering Atherosclerosis Study (CLAS)[27]	162	2
Familial Atherosclerosis Study (FATS)[28]	103	2.5
femoral artery disease Duffield et al.[29]	24	1.7

Fig. 77 Lipid modification with angiographic assessment.

treatment	lipid response (%)			reduction in CHD incidence (%)
	↓ chol	↓ TG	↑ HDL	
diet alone	13			23
clofibrate	9			20
cholestyramine	13			19
gemfibrozil	11	35	34	34
niacin	10			26
clofibrate + nicotinic acid	13	19		36

treatment	lipid response (%)			angiographic outcome (progression/regression)
	↓ chol	↓ TG	↑ HDL	
clofibrate + nicotinic acid	18	38	10	↓ progression
cholestyramine	15		8	↓ progression
colestipol + niacin	26		37	↓ progression 16% regression
colestipol + lovastatin	LDL ↓ 48		14	↓ progression >10% regression
colestipol + nicotinic acid	LDL ↓ 34		41	↓ progression >10% regression
cholestyramine nicotinic acid, or clofibrate	25	45	25	60% ↓ progression

Multiple risk factor intervention trials

Some of these trials have not shown greater reduction in CHD in the treatment group over the control group. This can be explained by:

● Failure to achieve significant improvement in risk factors, for example in the European Collaborative Trial.[30]

● Simultaneous improvement in the control group, in response to increased awareness of coronary risk factors during the course of the trial, for example in the MRFIT Study.[31]

However when risk factor improvement was greater in the treatment group, a reduction in CHD was observed, for example in the Oslo Study.[32]

THE OSLO STUDY				
no. in study	duration	treatment	response (% reduction)	% CHD reduction
1232	5 years	diet and anti-smoking advice	13 ↓ cholesterol 45 ↓ smoking 20 ↓ triglyceride	47 ↓ (myocardial infarction) (↓total mortality)

Fig. 78   Life table analysis of CHD (fatal and non-fatal myocardial infarction and sudden death) in intervention and control groups; the Oslo Study.[32]

Overall results of trials

The reduction in CHD due to lowering cholesterol is similar for diet or drug intervention as seen in an overview of the trials.

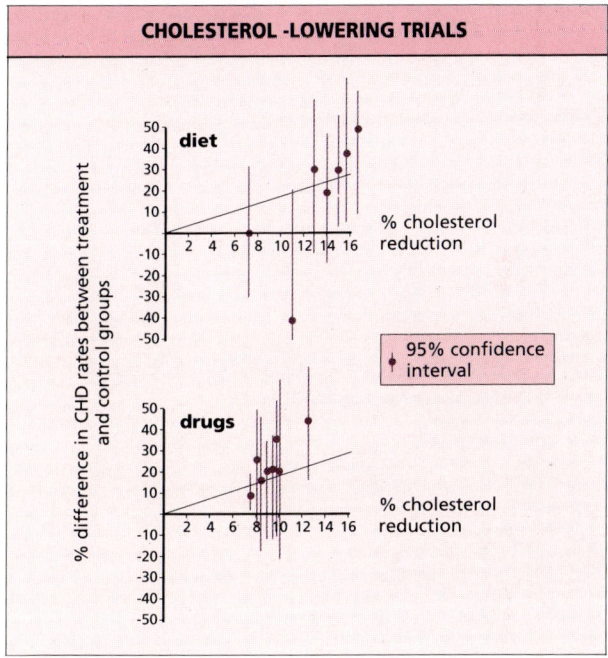

Fig. 79 Overall results of trials.

- A reduction of CHD by nearly a third can be achieved in less than 8 years.
- A 1% reduction in serum cholesterol is associated with 2% reduction in CHD risk.
- A 1% increase in HDL is associated with a 2–4% reduction in CHD risk.
- Triglyceride-lowering is associated with variable reductions in CHD risk.
- Effective lipid-lowering can slow the rate of progression and also achieve regression of atherosclerosis within 2 years.

MANAGEMENT OF LIPID DISORDERS

Management guidelines

Intervention is based on the following:
- Degree of elevation of serum cholesterol and/or triglyceride.
- Presence or absence of a personal history of coronary artery disease.
- Presence or absence of other CHD risk factors.

MANAGEMENT OF HYPERCHOLESTEROLAEMIA: EUROPEAN AND UK GUIDELINES		
cholesterol		assessment
mmol/l	mg/dl	
5.2–6.5	200–250	assess overall risk of CHD taking into account risk factors and younger age
6.5–7.8	250–300	assess overall risk of CHD, taking into account risk factors and younger age
>7.8	>300	assess overall risk of CHD, taking into account risk factors and younger age and consider referral to specialist clinic

Fig. 80 Summary of European[33] and UK[35] guidelines for management of hypercholesterolaemia. Intervention guidelines are based on total cholesterol levels and risk factor assessment.

RISK FACTORS
cigarette smoking
hypertension
diabetes mellitus
reduced HDL-cholesterol (HDL <0.9 mmol/l, 35 mg/al)
severe obesity
male
CHD in a first-degree relative under 55 years
previous stroke or peripheral vascular disease

Fig. 81 Risk factors in management of lipid disorders.[33,34]

management
correct overweight correct other modifiable risk factors advise dietary improvement
correct overweight correct other modifiable risk factors prescribe lipid-lowering diet drug treatment, if response inadequate and other risk factors present
correct overweight correct other modifiable risk factors prescribe lipid-lowering diet likely to require drug treatment

MANAGEMENT OF HYPERCHOLESTEROLAEMIA: USA GUIDELINES		
initial assessment	**management and follow-up**	
	total cholesterol mmol/l (mg/dl)	
without CHD and without 2 other risk factors	<5.2 (<200)	repeat total cholesterol within 5 years
	5.2–6.2 (200–239)	dietary information and recheck annually
with CHD or with 2 other CHD risk factors	5.2–6.2 (200–239)	lipoprotein analysis; then take further action based on LDL cholesterol levels
	≥6.2 (≥240)	
assessment	LDL cholesterol mmol/l (mg/dl)	**suggested treatment** / **minimum goal of therapy: LDL cholesterol mmol/l (mg/dl)**
without CHD and without 2 other risk factors	≥4.1 (≥160)	diet / <4.1 (<160)
	≥4.9 (≥190)	diet + drug / <4.1 (<160)
with CHD or with 2 other CHD risk factors	≥3.4 (≥130)	diet / <3.4 (<130)
	≥4.1 (≥160)	diet + drug / <3.4 (<130)

Fig. 82 Summary of USA guidelines[34] for management of hypercholesterolaemia. The guidelines are based on total cholesterol to assess risk, and on LDL-cholesterol to determine treatment and set therapeutic goals.

CAUSES AND MANAGEMENT OF HYPERTRIGLYCERIDAEMIA

causes	management recommendations	

obesity
alcohol excess
hypothyroidism
diabetes mellitus
renal disease
  (neophrotic
  syndrome,
  uraemia)
drugs: diuretics
  ß-blockers
  oestrogens
  retinoids
	initial
	management:
		identify and treat secondary
		causes

	drug
	therapy:
		controversial for borderline cases as
		  association of CHD and
		  hypertriglyceridaemia not
		  as strong as CHD and
		  hypercholesterolaemia
		recommended at TG
		  concentrations >6.0 mmol/l
		  if response to dietary
		  intervention is inadequate,
		  as the risk of pancreatitis is
		  increased

Fig. 83 Causes and management of secondary hypertriglyceridaemia.

MANAGEMENT OF HYPERTRIGLYCERIDAEMIA

triglyceride		assessment	management
mmol/l	mg/dl		

2.3–5.6	200–500	assess overall risk of
		CHD, taking into
		account risk factors
		and younger age.
		seek cause of raised TG
			correct overweight
			correct underlying
			  cause and risk factors
			prescribe lipid-
			  lowering diet
			monitor lipid levels

>5.6	>500	assess overall risk of
		CHD, taking into
		account risk factors
		and younger age
		
		seek cause of raised TG
		
		consider referral to
		specialist clinic
			likely to require drug
			  treatment
			correct overweight
			correct underlying
			  cause and risk factors
			prescribe lipid-
			  lowering diet

Fig. 84 Recommendations for management of hypertriglyceridae-mia. European[33,35] and USA[34] guidelines are similar.

| MANAGEMENT OF HYPERCHOLESTEROLAEMIA WITH HYPERTRIGLYCERIDAEMIA ||||
cholesterol mmol/l	triglyceride (mg/dl)	assessment	management
5.2–7.8 (200–300)	2.3–5.6 (200–500)	assess overall risk of CHD, taking into account risk factors and younger age.	correct overweight correct underlying cause and risk factors prescribe lipid-lowering diet drug treatment, if response inadequate and other risk factors present
		seek cause of raised lipids	
>7.8 (>300)	>5.6 (>500)	assess overall risk of CHD, taking into account risk factors and younger age	likely to require drug treatment correct overweight correct underlying cause and risk factors prescribe lipid-lowering diet
		seek cause of raised lipids	
		consider referral to specialist clinic	

Fig. 85 Recommendations for management of hypercholesterolaemia with hypertriglyceridaemia; elevation of both serum cholesterol and triglyceride (combined hyperlipidaemia) is a common disorder. UK,[35] European[33] and USA[34] guidelines are similar.

TARGET VALUES IN THE TREATMENT OF HYPERLIPIDAEMIA				
	no other CHD risk factors		multiple CHD risk factors	
	mmol/l	mg/dl	mmol/l	mg/dl
serum cholesterol	5.2–5.6	200–215	5.2	200
LDL-cholesterol	4.0	155	3.5	135
serum triglyceride	2.3	200	2.3	200

Fig. 86   Target values in the treatment of hyperlipidaemia (European guidelines[33]).

Diet

A reduction of total calories will reduce plasma triglycerides, and a reduction in dietary saturated fats and cholesterol will lower plasma cholesterol. Compliant patients can achieve a 20–25% reduction in plasma cholesterol, although there is considerable individual variation. Marked triglyceride reduction can be achieved when initial plasma triglyceride concentrations are high.

LIPID-LOWERING DIET: GENERAL ADVICE

1. Attain ideal body weight; reduce energy intake, or increase energy expenditure by exercise
2. Reduce total fat to ≤30% of total dietary energy intake.
3. Fat reduction: reduce saturated (mainly animal) fat to <10% of total energy
      partially replace saturated fat by monounsaturated and polyunsaturated fats (vegetable, olive and fish oils)
4. Reduce dietary cholesterol to <300 mg/day
5. Increase intake of complex carbohydrates and soluble fibres (fruit, cereals, vegetables)

Fig. 87   Lipid-lowering diet: general advice.

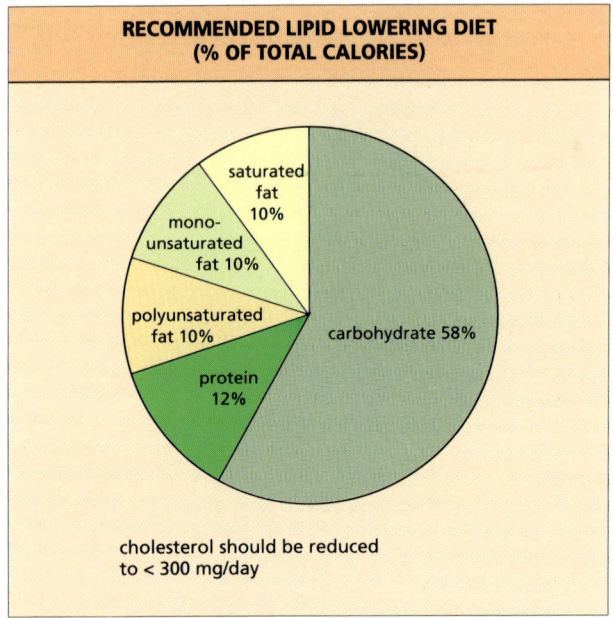

Fig. 88 Recommended lipid-lowering diet (% of total calories).

COMPOSITION OF FAT IN COMMON FOODS	
	% of saturated fat
dairy products	60
margarines (soft)	20–30
oils: coconut	75
corn, soya, olive	20
sunflower, safflower	15
meat: lamb	50
beef	45
pork	40
chicken	35
fish	20–25

Fig. 89 Composition of fat in common foods: foods with less saturated fat should be chosen.

SPECIFIC TRIGLYCERIDE-LOWERING DIETS
diet for endogenous hypertriglyceridaemia reduce calories to achieve ideal body weight avoid excessive carbohydrate and alcohol intake monounsaturated fats may be the main dietary fat
diet for chylomicronaemia syndrome restriction of saturated and unsaturated fats (total fat <10% of calories) medium-chain triglyceride supplements.

Fig. 90   Specific triglyceride-lowering diets.

Drugs
Drug therapy is generally recommended only when an appropriate diet has failed to reduce lipid levels sufficiently.

DRUG GROUPS USED FOR FAMILIAL LIPID DISORDERS	
disorder	**drug groups**
hypercholesterolaemia	bile acid sequestrants fibric acid derivatives nicotinic acid derivatives probucol HMG CoA reductase inhibitors
combined hyperlipidaemia	fibric acid derivatives nicotinic acid derivatives HMG CoA reductase inhibitors
endogenous hypertriglyceridaemia	fibric acid derivatives nicotinic acid derivatives fish oils (pharmacological doses)
apo E-2 homozygosity	fibric acid derivatives nicotinic acid derivatives

Fig. 91   Drug groups used for familial lipid disorders.

DRUG THERAPY FOR LIPID DISORDERS	
drug group + examples	**dosage range**
bile acid sequestrants	
cholestyramine	2–6 × 4 g
colestipol	2–6 × 5 g
fibric acid derivatives	
bezafibrate	3 × 200 mg or 1 × 400 mg
fenofibrate	3 × 100 mg or 1 × 250 mg
gemfibrozil	1–2 × 600 mg
HMG CoA reductase inhibitors	
lovastatin*	20–80 mg
pravastatin	10–40 mg
simvastatin	10–40 mg
nicotinic acid and derivatives	
nicotinic acid (niacin)	1–3 × 1–2 g
acipimox	1–3 × 250 mg
probucol	1–2 × 500 mg
fish oils	1–10 g
*not currently in UK	

Fig. 92 Drug therapy for lipid disorders.

TREATMENT FOR HOMOZYGOUS FAMILIAL HYPERCHOLESTEROLAEMIA	
treatment	**aim**
plasmapharesis (LDL-apharesis)	reduce LDL
liver transplantation	restore hepatic LDL receptors

Fig. 93 Treatment of homozygous familial hypercholesterolaemia.

adverse effects	contraindications
abdominal discomfort, constipation, diarrhoea, may decrease absorption of other drugs, triglyceride elevation	elevated plasma triglycerides, complete biliary obstruction, peptic ulcer, pregnancy
abdominal discomfort, nausea, rash, myalgia, may enhance effects of anticoagulants	severe liver or renal impairment, gallbladder disease, nephrotic syndrome, hypersensitivity, pregnancy
flatulence, raised liver & muscle enzymes ($\pm$ myopathy), rash	impairment of liver function, hypersensitivity, pregnancy, breast feeding
flushing, pruritus, nausea, glucose-intolerance (not observed with acipimox), dyspepsia, hyperuricaemia	impairment of liver function, congestive heart failure, recent myocardial infarction, gout, pregnancy, breast feeding, peptic ulcer, hypersensitivity
nausea, abdominal pain, prolong QT interval, sweat odour, rash	impairment of liver function, biliary obstruction, pregnancy, breast feeding, arrhythmia
nausea, flatulence	peptic ulcer

MONOTHERAPY				
	lipids (% change)		lipoproteins (% change)	
	cholesterol	triglyceride	LDL	HDL
bile acid sequestrants	15–30	5–30	15–30	3–8
fibric acid derivatives	10–20	30–50	20–25	10–25
HMG CoA reductase inhibitors	20–33	10–30	25–45	2–15
nicotinic acid and derivatives	15–30	20–60	15–40	10–20
probucol	5–15	0–5	8–15	10–25
fish oils	↑ variable ↓	10–60	↑ variable	5–10

increase   decrease   variable

Fig. 94 Expected changes (%) in lipids and lipoproteins at optimal dosage of a single drug (monotherapy).

DRUG COMBINATIONS	
drug combination	expected reduction in LDL-cholesterol (%)
bile acid sequestrant + nicotinic acid derivative	32–55
bile acid sequestrant + fibric acid derivative	25–40
bile acid sequestrant + probucol	25–40
bile acid sequestrant + HMG CoA reductase inhibitor	52–55
HMG CoA reductase inhibitor + nicotinic acid derivative	49–55
bile acid sequestrant + HMG CoA reductase inhibitor + nicotinic acid derivative	60–70

Fig. 95 Drug combinations. Cholesterol lowering can be greatly enhanced by using combinations of drugs that have different and complimentary mechanisms of action.

DETECTION AND LABORATORY INVESTIGATION OF LIPID DISORDERS

Approaches to detection

Population screening: the scale of the problems that would be encountered with this approach in order to provide advice, treatment and follow-up is illustrated by the prevalence of hypercholesterolaemia in, for example, the British population.

Opportunistic screening: measurement of lipids and assessment of other risk factors as part of routine medical practice.

Selective screening: aims to identify subjects with a high likelihood of a hyperlipidaemia, for example a family history of hyperlipidaemia or vascular disease, or cutaneous features of a lipid disorder and/or the presence of other risk factors.

PLASMA CHOLESTEROL LEVELS IN THE BRITISH POPULATION		
cholesterol mmol/l	mg/dl	% of population
>5.2	>200	63
>5.7	>220	45
>6.5	>250	25
>7.5	>290	3

Fig. 96 Plasma cholesterol levels in the British population.

RECOMMENDATIONS FOR INDIVIDUAL ASSESSMENT

history

personal history of hyperlipidaemia or CHD
  age of onset?
  treatment?

Family history of hyperlipidaemia, CHD or peripheral vascular disease
  in first-degree relative (parent or sibling)
  or second-degree relative
  age of onset?

known hypertension, diabetes mellitus, hypothyroidism?
alcohol consumption?
tobacco: number of cigarettes smoked? duration?
other medication?
current diet?

examination

weight
weight and height for body mass index (BMI) calculation
$$BMI = weight (kg) \div [height (m)]^2$$
blood pressure

corneal arcus, xanthelasmas, xanthomas (cutaneous, palmar,
  tendons)?

pulses
features of hypothyroidism, diabetes, etc.

laboratory investigation

fasting lipids: total cholesterol, TG and HDL

glucose
liver function test
γGT   to exclude/confirm
creatinine   secondary
urinary protein   hyperlipidaemia
thyroid function tests
haemoglobin blood count and film

Fig. 97   Recommendations for individual assessment.

Recommendations for laboratory measurement of lipids and lipoproteins

RECOMMENDATIONS: THE PATIENT

1. 12-h fast preferred but not essential for total or HDL cholesterol
2. Patient should be seated for at least 5 minutes
3. Avoid stasis (if needed a touriquet should be applied for the minimum of time)
4. Maintain habitual diet including alcohol—weight should be stable

defer: 2 weeks after minor illness
       2–3 months after myocardial infarction
       2–3 months after illness or pregnancy

a sample drawn within 24h of onset of mycocardial infarction may match the pre-infarction state
two measurements c. 1 month apart are required to reliably assess cholesterol status
serial measurements should be performed using the same laboratory

Fig. 98 Recommendations for laboratory measurement: the patient.

RECOMMENDATIONS: THE BLOOD SAMPLE

serum is preferred for lipid measurements
EDTA plasma (gives values 3% lower than serum) for lipoprotein fractionation

allow to clot in glass tubes for 30 min
separate serum or plasma within 3 h

store at: 4°C for up to 1 week,
         −20°C for up to 6 months.

Fig. 99 Recommendations for laboratory measurement: the blood sample.

Laboratory methods

Isolation of lipoproteins by ultracentrifugation or electrophoresis is time-consuming and expensive and not generally required in routine clinical investigation. Simpler measurements are preferred.

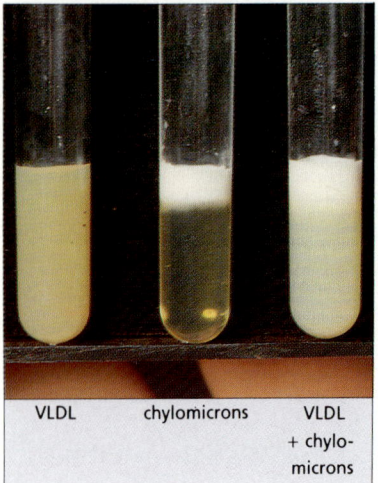

| VLDL | chylomicrons | VLDL + chylomicrons |

Fig. 100 Visual inspection of serum can determine the presence of chylomicrons in turbid fasting serum that has been stored refrigerated overnight. Chylomicrons float to the surface of the serum, forming a milky layer. VDLs also cause turbidity in plasma but, being of greater density, they do not 'float' on storage.

MEASUREMENT OF LIPIDS, LIPOPROTEINS AND APOPROTEINS

lipid/lipoprotein	method
cholesterol triglyceride	simple enzymic techniques
HDL-cholesterol	measurement in plasma following precipitation of other lipoproteins
LDL-cholesterol (not valid in presence of chylomicrons, IDL or TG >4.6 mmol/l, 410 mg/dl)	use Friedwald equation: $$LDL = \text{total chol} - \left(HDL\text{-chol} + \frac{TG}{2.19}\right) \text{ mmol/l}$$ $$LDL = \text{total chol} - \left(HDL\text{-chol} + \frac{TG}{5.0}\right) \text{ mg/dl}$$
apo A apo B Lp(a)	radio-immunoassay and non-isotopic immunoassay techniques

Fig. 101 Measurements of lipids, lipoproteins and apoproteins. Measurement of HDL is also useful to identify individuals with a minor elevation of total cholesterol due to borderline elevation of HDL.

DIAGNOSTIC TESTS PERFORMED IN SPECIALIST LABORATORIES

test	disorder
apo E–2 phenotyping	apo E–2 homozygosity
apo C-II phenotyping	chylomicronaemia
post-heparin LPL activity	lipoprotein lipase deficiency
LDL receptor activity	familial hypercholesterolaemia

Fig. 102 Diagnostic tests performed only by specialist laboratories.

REFERENCES

1. Assmann G. Lipid Metabolism and Atherosclerosis. Stuttgart: F.K.Schattauer Verlag GmbH, 1982.

2. Mann JI, Lewis B, Shepherd J, et al. Blood lipid concentrations and other cardiovascular risk factors: distribution, prevalence, and detection in Britain. Br Med J 1988; 296: 1702–1706.

3. Brown MS, Goldstein JL. Receptor-mediated endocytosis: insights from the lipoprotein receptor system. Proc Natl Acad Sci USA 1979; 76: 3330–3337.

4. Ross R, Glomset JA. The pathogenesis of atherosclerosis. N Engl J Med 1976; 295: 369.

5. Keys A. Seven countries. A multivariate analysis of death and coronary heart disease. Cambridge, Massachusetts: Harvard University Press, 1980.

6. Nichamen MZ, Hamilton HB, Kagan A, Grier T, Sacks T, Syme SL. Epidemiological studies of coronary heart disease and stroke in Japanese men living in Japan, Hawaii and California: distribution of biochemical risk factors. Am J Epidemiol 1975; 102: 491–501.

7. Martin MJ, Hulley SB, Browner WS, Kuller LH, Wentworth D. Serum cholesterol blood pressure and mortality: implications from a cohort of 361 662 men. Lancet 1986; ii: 933–936.

8. Stamler J, Wentworth D, Neaton J. Is the relationship between serum cholesterol and risk of death from coronary heart disease continuous and graded? JAMA 1986; 256: 2823–2828.

9. Shaper AG, Pocock SJ, Walker M, Phillips AN, Whitehead TP, MacFarlane PW. Risk factors for ischaemic heart disease: the prospective phases of the British Regional Heart Study. J Epidem Comm Health 1985; 39: 197–209.

10. Gordon T, Castelli WP, Hjortland MC, Kannel WB, Dawber TR. High density lipoprotein as a protective factor against coronary heart disease: The Framingham study. Am J Med 1977; 62: 707–714.

11. Gordon DJ, Probstfield JL, Garrison RJ, et al. High density lipoprotein cholesterol and cardiovascular disease: four prospective American studies. Circulation 1989; 79: 8–15.

12. Gordon DJ, Knoke J, Probstfield JL, et al (for the Lipid Research Clinics Program). High density lipoprotein cholesterol and coronary heart disease in hypercholesterolemic men: The Lipid Research Clinics Coronary Primary Prevention Trial. Circulation 1986; 74: 1217–1225.

13. Watkins LO, Neaton JD, Kuller LH (for the MRFIT Research Group). Racial differences in high-density lipoprotein cholesterol and coronary heart disease incidence in the usual-care

group of the Multiple Risk Factor Intervention Trial. Am J Cardiol 1986; 57: 538–545.

14. Assmann G, Schulte H, Oberwittler W, Hauss WH. New aspects in the prediction of coronary artery disease: The Prospective Cardiovascular Münster study. In: Fidge NH, Nestel PJ (eds) Proceedings of the 7th International Atherosclerosis Symposium. Amsterdam: Elsevier, 1986: 19–24.

15. Pocock SJ, Shaper AG, Phillips AN. Concentrations of high density lipoprotein cholesterol, triglycerides, and total cholesterol in ischaemic heart disease. Br Med J 1989; 298: 998–1002.

16. Goldbourt U, Holtzman E, Neufeld HN. Total and high density lipoprotein cholesterol in the serum and risk of mortality: evidence of a threshold effect. Br Med J 1985; 290: 1239–1243.

17. Miller NE, Thelle DS, Forde OH, Mjos OD. The Tromso Heart Study. High-density lipoprotein and coronary heart disease: a case-control study. Lancet 1977; i: 965–968.

18. Enger SC, Hjermann I, Foss OP, et al. High-density lipoprotein cholesterol and myocardial infarction and sudden coronary death: a prospective case-control study in middle-aged men of the Oslo study. Artery 1979; 5: 170–181.

19. Dayton S, Pearce ML, Hashimoto S, Dixon WJ, Tomiyasu U. A controlled clinical trial of a diet high in unsaturated fat in preventing complications of atherosclerosis. Circulation 1969; 39, 40 (suppl. II): 1–63.

20. Oliver MF, Heady JA, Morris JN, Cooper J. A co-operative trial in the primary prevention of ischaemic heart disease using clofibrate. Report from the Committee of Principal Investigators. Br Heart J 1978; 40: 1069–1118.

21. Lipid Research Clinics Program. The lipid research clinics coronary primary prevention trial results: I. Reduction in incidence of coronary heart disease. JAMA 1984; 251: 351–364.

22. Frick MH, Elo O, Haapa K et al. Helsinki heart study: primary-prevention trial with gemfibrozil in middle-aged men with dyslipidemia. N Engl J Med 1987; 317: 1237–1245.

23. The Coronary Drug Project Research Group. Clofibrate and niacin in coronary heart disease. JAMA 1975; 231: 360–381.

24. Carlson LS, Rosenhamer G. Reduction of mortality in the Stockholm Ischaemic Heart Disease Secondary Prevention Study by combined treatment with clofibrate and nicotinic acid. Acta Med Scand 1988; 223: 405–418.

25. Nikkila EQ, Viikinkoski P, Valle M. Effect of lipid lowering treatment on progression of coronary atherosclerosis. A 7-year prospective angiographic study. Circulation 1983; 68 (suppl. III): 111–188.

26. Levy RI, Brensike JF, Epstein SE, et al. The influence of changes in lipid values induced by cholestyramine and diet on progression of coronary artery disease: results of the NHLBI type II coronary intervention study. Circulation 1984; 69: 325–337.

27. Blankenhorn DH, Nessim SA, Johnson RL, Sanmarco ME, Azen SP, Cashen-Hemphill L. Beneficial effects of combined colestipol–niacin therapy on coronary atherosclerosis and coronary venous bypass grafts. JAMA 1987; 257: 3233–3240.

28. Greg Brown B, Lin JT, Schaefer SM, Kaplan CA, Dodge HT, Albers JJ. Niacin or lovastatin, combined with colestipol, regress coronary atherosclerosis and prevent clinical events in men with elevated apolipoprotein B. Circulation 1989; 80: 1061 (Abstr.).

29. Duffield RGM, Lewis B, Miller NE, Jamieson CW, Brunt JNH, Colchester ACF. Treatment of hyperlipidaemia retards progression of symptomatic femoral atherosclerosis. Lancet 1983; ii: 639–642.

30. World Health Organization European Collaborative Group. European Collaborative Trial of Multifactorial Prevention of Coronary Heart Disease: final report on the 6-year results. Lancet 1986: i: 869–872.

31. Multiple Risk Factor Intervention Trial Research Group. Multiple Risk Factor Intervention Trial: risk factor changes and mortality results. JAMA 1982; 248: 1465.

32. Hjermann I, Velve Byre K, Holme I, Leren P. Effect of diet and smoking intervention on the incidence of coronary heart disease. Report from the Oslo Study Group of a randomised trial in healthy men. Lancet 1981; ii: 1303–1310.

33. European Atherosclerosis Society. The recognition and management of hyperlipidaemia in adults: a policy statement of the European Atherosclerosis Society. Eur Heart J 1988; 9: 571–600.

34. Report of the National Cholesterol Education Program Expert Panel on Detection, Evaluation, and Treatment of High Blood Cholesterol in Adults. Arch Intern Med 1988; 148: 36–69.

35. British Hyperlipidaemia Association. Strategies for reducing coronary heart disease and desirable limits for blood lipid concentrations: guidelines of the British Hyperlipidaemia Association. Br Med J 1987; 295: 1245–1246.

INDEX